HYSTERECTOMY: WOMAN TO WOMAN

SUE ELLEN BARBER

BookPartners, Inc.
Wilsonville, Oregon

All information in this book is based on the experiences and research of the author. This information is shared with the understanding that you accept complete responsibility for your own health and well-being. Any attempt to diagnose and treat an illness should come under the direction of a physician.

BookPartners, Inc.
P. O. Box 922
Wilsonville, Oregon 97070

To Mom and Dad (I miss you, Dad!)
and most especially
to my Honey

Acknowledgments

So many have contributed so much, and I am grateful to all for their assistance and encouragement. This project would not have been possible without them.

Special thanks go to the women who talked so freely about their own experiences, as well as my family and friends. Also to Thorn and Ursula Bacon, Dr. Raymond E. Barber, Patrice Butkiewicz, Dr. Lillian Dyson, Dr. Brian Guz, Dr. Don K. Harrison, Wendy Miller, Sally LePla-Perry, Mary Lou Slater, Dr. Margaret A. Szymanski, my son and daughter, my grandboys, and my mom.

Table Of Contents

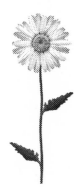

Prologue –

The Why And How Of This Book.

~ ~

These pages discuss the most basic physical alteration a woman can experience.

Hysterectomy

My intent is to provide a balanced presentation that considers this complex issue from all sides — before, during and after surgery takes place. By subject matter and tonality, I am addressing women in this work.

But the book is also for those who love us, and those who care for our health and well-being. It is my hope that our husbands, lovers, companions, friends, children, and yes, even our gynecologists, will find information of interest in these pages. Despite the fairly typical male reaction of my brother (a highly skilled, well-travelled Ph.D.) to the news I was working on this volume —

"Obviously you don't expect men to read it!" — this is an opportunity for those closest to us — *even men* — to better understand one of the most personal and fundamental experiences a woman can have.

WHAT AND WHY

Hysterectomy goes to the very foundation of what makes us the female of the species. The female reproductive system defines our anatomy, regulates our temperament, modulates our sex drive, influences our health — in short, governs every aspect of our lives.

Yet more than 600,000 American women part with this defining organ every year.

Including me.

The official name for what I had done is "total abdominal hysterectomy with bilateral salpingo-oophorectomy with anterior repair" — "TAHBSO with anterior repair" is the medical shorthand. Translated, it means that via abdominal incision, my gynecologist removed my uterus (total abdominal hysterectomy), both fallopian tubes (bilateral salpingo) and ovaries (oophorectomy). When she was finished, the urologist took over and performed a bladder suspension. That's the anterior repair part.

The removal of my female apparatus was necessitated by severe fibroids — the type that caused four-week long periods, heavy bleeding, large blood clots, anemia, and a long list of other complications and compromises.

By the time I had the surgery, these insidious, unwelcome and little-understood fibroid growths had affected

~ ~

virtually every aspect of my lifestyle. I decided to add a bladder suspension to the operation because for years I had not been able to walk down the street and sneeze without stopping to cross my legs.

Much to my surprise, having a hysterectomy was not simply a matter of checking into the hospital, undergoing the procedure, resting up for a few days and getting with business as usual.

In part that resulted from my never having had major surgery before; I simply did not know what to expect.

But I believe it also has to do with a lack of *real* information about this surgery and how it affects a woman. Having a hysterectomy is, in many regards, a life-altering experience.

During the decision-making phase I tried to make sense out of such contradictory assertions as 90 percent of hysterectomies are unnecessary and 95 percent of women who have the surgery report they would undergo the procedure again if circumstances were the same. Meanwhile, the reality of a cost-driven medical establishment often produced hurried office visits and unsatisfying answers to my most basic questions.

Over and over I wondered as I wrestled with my situation: where was the specific, reasonable, personalized information I needed to make intelligent, informed choices about *me?*

Once I had actually decided to have a hysterectomy, I again searched in vain, this time for detailed descriptions of what surgery and recovery would actually be like.

~ ~

The simple fact was: I couldn't find the hysterectomy experience, in its entirety, beginning to end, discussed anywhere, at least not from the perspective of a woman who has been there.

That is why I want to share in these pages what has happened to me.

Actually, my operation was somewhat different from the typical hysterectomy in three regards. First, I was several years older, at 50, than the 42-1/2 which is the average age of women having a hysterectomy. Second, my surgery went beyond the basics with the inclusion of the oophorectomy and the bladder suspension. The third difference was impossible to address in any quantifiable manner: I am single, whereas most women who have hysterectomies are married. There simply was no source to help me assess what effect a hysterectomy might have on my intimate life. Which is not to say that married women are any less concerned than I was about the implications of the surgery on their relationships. All of us, no matter what our marital or relationship status may be, must address the issue of how a hysterectomy might impact these crucial aspects of our lives.

MY APPROACH

What we have here is my account of a personal odyssey. Talking about so personal and intimate an experience will, of necessity, expose aspects of my physical and psychological landscape, as well as my lifestyle. So be it,

~ ~ ~ ~ ~ ~ ~ ~ ~ ~ ~ ~ ~ ~ ~ ~ ~ ~ ~ ~

especially if my descriptions lend assistance to others who may find themselves on a similar journey.

To make the book as useful as possible, I have included discussions of everything from the controversy surrounding this surgery to practical tips on how to cope with the hospital stay to what it feels like to resume having sex.

In order to be more comprehensive, several "About ..." sections accompany the narrative. These are brief descriptions presenting facts and data from a medical perspective about various topics associated with hysterectomy.

Finally, I have concluded each chapter by summarizing "What Was Important" at that point in the process, in the form of words of advice.

I must emphasize that I am not a medical professional, and this book is, in no way, intended to be a scientific study. While I have reviewed a number of sources on the subject, I make no claim to having conducted an exhaustive search of the literature. There is no random sample and no statistical analysis. This book is anecdotal, an oral history — just me and a number of other women talking in a very personal manner about this important event in our lives.

A word of warning: parts of this narrative are graphic and candid. That is intentional, because I want to convey a realistic sense of what women may experience. Other accounts are intensely personal. Including such details was also a conscious choice on my part, since having a hysterectomy affects the most intimate aspects of our lives. For that reason, and once again, to protect privacy, I have assigned everyone involved names other than their own. I have done the same with my doctors. Let me state that I have the utmost respect for and confidence in them and their professional capabilities and abilities. But our consultations took place in the privacy of the examining room, and I decided the sanctity of physician/patient privilege must be observed. Although some compression of events occurs, of necessity, in the telling, be assured that every incident I describe, and every conversation, is genuine and reported as factually and faithfully as possible.

MY PURPOSE

By compiling these experiences, I want to provide a useful handbook that informs women as they negotiate the many intricacies of hysterectomy.

Although the physical aspects of the surgery are fairly straightforward, it is the psychological and emotional effects and ramifications that are less well-defined, more troublesome and ultimately, the most important. Physically, our bodies generally recover from the trauma of surgery. But what happens to us in toto is an area that is just now being explored.

This fact is, many women undergo this operation, and we deserve to know more about it and what to expect. By speaking openly, freely, and at length about the details, we can put the experience in perspective. And despite considerable debate, this surgery may actually be beneficial, under appropriate circumstances, as a means of improving the quality of our lives.

~ ~ ~ ~ ~ ~ ~ ~ ~ ~ ~ ~ ~ ~ ~ ~ ~ ~ ~ ~

That brings me back to the fundamental purpose of this book. For women who are contemplating this surgery, recovering from it, or simply seeking more information, I hope to lessen the feeling of isolation many of us encounter. By talking about the entire, extended process of hysterectomy, I wish to help women, and those who love us and take care of us, approach this experience in all its manifestations and ramifications.

To all women, I want to offer a sense of support and hope.

Part I

How To Decide

Having a hysterectomy is a fundamental life choice. These chapters explore what goes into making a decision and provide advice on how to prepare for surgery.

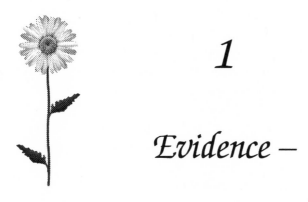

1

Evidence –

Gathering The Data

~ ~

Brisk and clear, with temperatures around 20 degrees and bright winter sunshine overhead. Northern Michigan had presented us with a glorious day for crosscountry skiing. Trail conditions were invigorating — perfectly groomed tracks that twisted uphill and down, through the vivid green of forests where the only sound was a slight, sighing breeze.

I was skiing hard and had been for an hour or so. What a pleasure to be out of the office, in the fresh air, challenging my body for a change, instead of just my brain! I was on the longest loop around the outskirts of the resort property, fifteen kilometers from our condo, enjoying a winter weekend in February.

Another hill coming up — not too long, but steep. Time for a little more power to the legs, dig in the arms harder, up and over....

Damn!

Of course, I knew immediately what the warm gush between my legs meant: I had soaked through the ultra-super tampon I was wearing and blood was running onto the heavy-duty sanitary napkin. I had put on fresh supplies just before hitting the trail, so I skied on. Sometimes, I knew from long experience with heavy periods, the gushing meant a blood clot had passed and soon the flow would back off.

Not this time. The hot sensation continued, until I was worried the blood would overflow the pad and start down the legs of my ski suit.

Remembering the extra tampon I had stuck in the pocket of my ski jacket, just in case, I began looking around for a bit of privacy. Plenty of trees, but I would have to take my skis off to navigate far enough into the woods to get out of view of other skiers. With two feet of snow on the ground, I did not relish the thought of sinking in up to my knees.

Finally, I spotted a hut — a rest room, actually, since this area was a golf course in the summertime. I headed toward the structure. Of course, it was locked.

More blood; I could feel it warm and insistent. I had two choices: try to ski back to the condo, although I was a long way out, and by this point I was worried about leaving drops of red behind me on the trail. Or, I could change the tampon.

I opted for the latter. Maneuvering to the side of the hut where I was more or less out of sight, I started taking off

~ ~

layers. Gloves first, then jacket; unzip my one-piece lycra ski suit from the neck (great attire for skiing, tough to get out of quickly); pull off the sleeves, next the long underwear, panties, finally down to where I needed to be.

In the shade of the hut the temperature was about 10 degrees. I was so numb by the time I replaced the tampon I could barely accomplish the business at hand. I did not have another pad, so I had to leave the old one in place and hope for the best. Shivering, I replaced my clothing.

Now, what to do with the soiled material? I did not want to drop it in the snow where I stood and let someone else come upon this unpleasant residue. Putting it in my pocket, even wrapped in a tissue, would result in a bloody mess. I finally decided the best of several bad possibilities was to throw it as far as I could down the hill and into the woods.

I did, and nearly followed it when I slipped on the ice.

That night at dinner I told Kal, my boyfriend and weekend companion, that I was seriously rethinking the hysterectomy question.

FACTS AND CONTROVERSY

A woman who must face the hysterectomy choice is swirled by a dilemma that ultimately comes down to a very personal issue: How do I make an intelligent, informed decision about *my* body?

Undertaking a serious consideration of hysterectomy requires an examination of a complex and confusing web of medical, personal, emotional, familial, sexual, professional, social and financial factors, to name just some of the things we have to think about. Few clear-cut answers exist for any of these issues, but they form the context within which the decision to have this surgery must be made.

Let's start with the controversy surrounding hysterectomy, because women contemplating the surgery, including me, would find it difficult not to be confused. We are bombarded by contentious debate taking place in medical circles, books, magazines, newspapers and television talk shows; intelligent, dispassionate discussion, on the other hand, may be difficult to find.

An often-cited rule of thumb for any operation is that it should be performed after nonsurgical treatments have failed, and then only if it can prolong life and has a reasonable chance of success. Hysterectomy can meet the "easy chance of success" part of the equation. Although regarded as major surgery, from the medical point of view the operation is relatively easy to perform and generally leads to few long-term complications. It is the "failure of nonsurgical treatments" and "prolonging life" part of the formula that get very murky, very fast.

The fact is, only 10 to 15 percent of hysterectomies are performed in cases of malignancy, precancerous conditions, or other life-threatening circumstances, including emergencies during or after childbirth and for some types of pelvic inflammatory disease. The remaining 85 to 90 percent of hysterectomies fall in the "to relieve symptoms" category. These are discretionary surgeries, done in response to lifestyle considerations, leading physicians, policy makers, patients, advocates, feminists and others into a noisy discussion about the necessity and advisability of hysterectomy. The squabbling has gone on for fifty years.

~ ~

Which leads to the fundamental question: Why would I, or any otherwise healthy woman, willfully agree to being sliced open and having the female part of her insides abruptly, albeit skillfully, cut out?

A number of observers have argued that to do so would be absolute lunacy on my part.

"Curing a pelvic disease with a hysterectomy is the equivalent of treating a mild headache with decapitation," warned Dr. Francis L. Hutchins, Jr., Director of Gynecology and Women's Services at Graduate Hospital in Philadelphia. (cited by Arnot, *Good Housekeeping,* January 1993)

Dr. Stanley West, head of Reproductive Endocrinology at St. Vincent's Hospital, declares that hysterectomy is big business, and medically necessary only in cases of malignancy. *(The Hysterectomy Hoax)*

Nora W. Coffey, executive director of the Hysterectomy Education Resources and Services (HERS) Foundation, who described herself as "hysterectomized and castrated" following removal of her uterus and ovaries, goes even further. She contends it is impossible for a woman to be the same following removal of her sexual and reproductive organs. "Under what circumstances would a doctor say to a man, 'You're not having any more children, so what do you need your penis and testicles for?' Even a man who was a hundred years old would never consent to having his sexual and reproductive organ removed unless it was to save his life." (cited by Wiltz, *Essence,* October 1992)

Still, there is no scarcity of women who have consented to the removal of their uterus. Fully one third (some estimates say 37 percent) of American women undergo a hysterectomy by the time they are 65.

Estimates of the number of surgeries performed annually in the United States, vary, with different sources citing numbers ranging from 500,000 to 700,000. Based on hospital records, indications are that the overall rate has somewhat declined in the past two decades, from more than 800,000 surgeries per year in the mid 1970s, to the best-guess figure of 600,000 today. Research does show that the rate of hysterectomies varies by region, with more surgeries performed in the South than in other areas of the country. Also, more hysterectomies are performed in the United States than in Europe, for reasons that are not clear and apparently have not been subjected to serious study.

Are doctors getting rich by duping unsuspecting women into having hysterectomies, as some critics charge? Or, do they continue to subscribe to outmoded thinking about common gynecological problems, as other observers maintain?

Hysterectomy is undeniably big business, generating an estimated $4 billion annually for the medical industry. It is the second most frequently performed surgical procedure for women (Cesarean sections ranking first). In the recent past, the surgery was considered an easy cure-all for bothersome female problems; indeed, women over the age of forty routinely had the surgery on the advice it was time to "join the club." Often these women had the operation for reasons that were not clearly explained and that they did not understand. Without a doubt, that still goes on, as does the debate about when hysterectomy may be advisable. Various studies have concluded that 27 percent *(Consumer Reports,* July 1992), 33 percent (Blue Cross/Blue Shield of Illinois in a 1990 study), or 41 percent (RAND Corporation in a 1993 study) of these operations are unwarranted or questionable.

~ ~

Unfortunately, the whole subject lends itself to confusion, in part because the considerations involved in having a hysterectomy are seldom easy delineations of black and white.

Absent a life-threatening illness, hysterectomy is nearly always an elective procedure, done to improve the quality of a woman's life.

The fundamental issue becomes how to define or quantify something so intangible and individual as "quality of life."

The most common conditions leading to hysterectomy, according to the Maine Women's Health Study (1994), are fibroids (30–35 percent), abnormal bleeding (20–22 percent), chronic pelvic pain (15–18 percent), endometriosis (10 percent), uterine prolapse (5–10 percent), precancerous conditions such as cervical intraepithelial neoplasia and endometrial hyperplasia (8–10 percent), and other diagnoses (2 percent). Frequently, various combinations of these conditions are present in a single woman, as was true in my case. The symptoms resulting from these various conditions can vary widely, ranging from none to quite severe.

Determining if, and when, a hysterectomy is appropriate becomes highly problematic. Despite the fact that this surgery is a major, monumental, irreversible life decision, there is no clear set of cause-and-effect guidelines to help us in making a decision.

In the absence of such data, I decided the logical place to start was with an honest assessment of my medical situation. A long litany of classic symptoms — heavy bleeding, clotting, cramps, prolonged periods, spotting, anemia —

finally forced me to make a determination about the effect of my female problems on the overall quality of my life.

ABOUT FEMALE REPRODUCTIVE ANATOMY

The reproductive system consists of an extremely complicated group of organs that interact in a number of ways.

The two ovaries are walnut-sized organs responsible for producing the hormones that regulate every aspect of a woman's body. They also house hundreds of unfertilized eggs.

Connected to each ovary is a fallopian tube. The tube is about four inches long and leads from the ovaries to the uterus.

The uterus is an upside-down, pear-shaped organ three to four inches long and weighing two to three ounces. The inner walls of this thick, muscular organ are lined with tissue called the endometrium.

The lowermost portion of the uterus is the cervix, opening into the vagina.

The vagina is a three-to-four-inch long canal connecting the cervix to the outside of the body.

A series of ligaments attach the uterus and vagina to the pelvic wall.

The entire structure nestles in the lower part of the abdomen, with the bladder in front of and below the uterus, and the rectum behind.

At the beginning of each menstrual cycle, the ovaries release the hormone estrogen to prepare the uterine lining for a possible pregnancy. One ovary releases an egg into the fallopian tube, where it travels to the uterus. If the egg is not fertilized, the

~ ~

endometrium is discharged during the monthly period. When a woman enters menopause, typically between the ages of 45 and 55, the ovaries gradually stop releasing eggs and cease producing estrogen. Periods become irregular, eventually stopping altogether.

PERSONAL BACKGROUND

Let me say that I am not someone who avoids doctors and hospitals. I have enough sense to take care of myself, especially as it relates to regular mammograms, breast and pelvic exams, pap smears, and similar female concerns.

Although no athlete, I exercise regularly, with a combination of running, swimming, aerobics and in season, bicycling and crosscountry skiing. I try to eat sensibly (low fat, lots of pasta, grains, fish, fruits and vegetables), and drink alcohol in moderation. I enjoy my family, the company of friends and am blessed to be in a strong relationship with a wonderful man.

By way of brief background: I am a lifelong Midwesterner and a college graduate with a Master's degree. I am an advertising and marketing writer by profession. Although I have been married, I am a long-time single-again, having raised two children on my own, and am the adoring grandmother to two boisterous preschool boys.

For years I also had fibroids, which is what led to that proverbial "ah ha!" moment. Freezing my butt off in February in the woods, I finally said to myself, "This is dumb!"

~ ~

ABOUT FIBROIDS

The uterine tumors commonly called "fibroids" are more properly known in medical terminology as leiomyomas, fibromyomas or myomas. These balls of muscular and connective tissue, which have their own blood supply, develop from the cells that make up the muscle of the uterus and can form and grow in a number of locations — inside the uterus, on the organ's outer surface and within the muscles of the uterine wall. They can also be attached to the uterus by a stemlike structure or appear in various combinations of the above. Fibroids can range in size from pea-like growths to masses as large as a soccer ball. They can distort the uterus, swell it to the size of a multi-month pregnancy and put pressure on adjacent organs such as the bladder and bowel. In some cases, they can fill the entire abdomen.

That fibroids are quite common is borne out by the statistics: From 25 to 40% of Caucasian women develop fibroids, while estimates for African American women run as high as 75%. Estrogen appears to affect fibroids; they tend to grow larger with increased estrogen levels and frequently shrink when estrogen diminishes, as during menopause.

Little is known about why fibroids develop or why they are more common among black women than white. The knots of tissue appear most often when women are in the their late 30s or early 40s, although they can show up in teenagers. Often, they enlarge over the years. Development appears to be related to a genetic predisposition, which means that fibroids are influenced by heredity and tend to run in families.

~ ~

Women who begin menstruating early, before age 11 or 12, seem to be more likely to have fibroids and develop them at an earlier age; they are also more common among women who have not had children. Being overweight seems to increase the risk as well. There is some evidence that fibroids are related to hypertension, which could, to an extent, account for the higher incidence among African Americans — high blood pressure is a common problem for blacks. A few medical professionals and other advocates, especially those who take a holistic approach to health, attribute fibroids to nutritional and emotional issues, relating their development to poor diet, childhood stress or unresolved anger and fear.

For some women, fibroids are completely asymptomatic; even large growths may cause no discomfort or abnormal bleeding. Many other women, however, exhibit a variety of symptoms, often in combination: heavy, frequent bleeding; clotting; cramping; fatigue; anemia; abdominal or lower back pain; pain during sex; pressure resulting in frequent urination and/or bowel problems; infertility and miscarriages.

Despite the fact that fibroids are nearly always benign (less than 1% of fibroids become cancerous), other complications occasionally develop. For example, they may fill with calcium deposits and become visible on x-rays. They may outgrow their blood supply or twist on their stalk, causing gangrene due to loss of blood supply. If located near the fallopian tubes or cervix, they may obstruct the uterus, with infertility the result.

NOT A NEW PROBLEM

Actually my condition had begun to manifest itself years before the crosscountry skiing episode. As long ago as 1986, I remember hiking on magnificent Mt. Rainier in Washington State, well above timberline, and desperately searching for a big rock. I was out hiking, experiencing one of my usual heavy periods. I thought I had protected myself adequately by inserting two tampons and putting on a double layer of sanitary napkins before I left my room. Not so. After a couple hours of tramping up the trail, I was forced by the all-too-familiar feel of gushing blood to look around for a place to change pads and tampons, out of the view of fellow hikers. What else was I supposed to do when I was bleeding faster than I could get back to the lodge?

At that point, I attributed my bleeding to a pattern that had begun at age twelve, when I first started menstruating. My periods always seemed to last longer and require more pads than those of other girls. Later, during the years I took birth control pills, my periods were regulated and blessedly light. Once I reached forty, however, and was told I was too old to take the pills, my pattern of long, heavy periods not only reappeared, it got worse. At the same time, I was becoming aware of other differences in my body; I figured it was all part of the onset of my change of life.

The official diagnosis of my fibroids came in 1989. The discovery was typical: during a routine check-up I described my heavy periods. When the doctor did a pelvic exam, she noted my uterus was enlarged, and suggested that a fibroid was the probable culprit. A subsequent visit to the gynecologist and an ultrasound confirmed the suspicion.

~ ~

After that, the evidence that finally led me to hysterectomy began to accumulate.

The Red Cross turndowns, for example. I have been a regular blood donor for a number of years, especially since my father died of leukemia. (Figuring a lot of nice people helped him by donating, I felt the least I could do was assist somebody else's dad.) But by 1990 I was occasionally getting rejected as a donor. A check of my hemoglobin, which is standard Red Cross procedure before accepting a donation, would indicate my red blood count was abnormally low and I was anemic. This did not happen all the time, but there was a pattern — always after a period.

Memorial Day 1991 was a prime instance of my bleeding playing havoc with my plans. It was supposed to be a pleasant weekend spent with friends at a lakefront cottage. Except I was having a period, a very bad one. For three solid days, I monopolized the only bathroom, frequently filling and emptying the waste basket with soaked and discarded sanitary pads and tampons. Because I quickly ran through what I had thought before leaving home would be adequate supplies, I had to make a hasty late-night run to the nearest convenience store and pay exorbitantly for more. My friends began wondering about me. My hostess and close friend Ann, sympathized, knowing I was tender with cramps, plagued by heavy flow and generally miserable.

Romantic weekends? My periods always seemed to coincide perfectly with such plans. I did learn one trick to salvage at least a shred of dignity — if I was not flowing too heavily, I could insert a birth control sponge to soak up and hold back the blood, still allowing decent and unmessy sex. (Unfortunately, sponges are no longer available, further limiting our already woefully inadequate birth control choices — but that's another story.) A diaphragm also works to hold back the blood, although it was always difficult for me to use one because of the increasingly distorted shape of my uterus and its tipped-back position in my body cavity.

Client meetings often became an embarrassment. I attended such sessions clutching, as discreetly as possible, my bag full of supplies. Suit pockets held a couple tampons, but they were not large enough for super, extra-long pads, or enough plugs to get through a four-hour meeting. A useful strategy I developed for concealing extra pads was to stash them in my bra. One especially difficult incident occurred when I was on the road, rehearsing executives of a major international company for speeches they were to make at a convention. Fortunately, none of their presentations was more than twenty minutes long, which was about how often I had to excuse myself to visit the ladies' room, my bag of bulky supplies tucked under one arm. I needed to give full attention to the rehearsals; instead, my concentration was divided between what my clients were saying and the bloody, crampy distraction gushing from my body.

And there were always blood clots — big, ugly masses of tissue that looked like liver — oozing out of me. I could always tell when I was passing a large one; my uterus contracted with labor-like pains. I remember, on one unpleasant occasion, getting out of the shower, and discharging a four-inch long mass that slid right past the tampon I was wearing (a super, of course) and dropped at my feet, quivering, on the bathroom floor.

My periods typically lasted 10 to 12 days, starting with spotting for three or four days, progressing to very

~ ~ ~ ~ ~ ~ ~ ~ ~ ~ ~ ~ ~ ~ ~ ~ ~ ~ ~ ~

heavy bleeding and clotting for the next four days or so, and then spotting for another several days. (No wonder romantic weekends were merely a fantasy — I was bleeding all the time!) After 15 days, maybe 20, the cycle would start again.

I was constantly checking my underwear for spotting. Sometimes the blood would start abruptly, so that I began wearing a light pad even between periods. Eventually, every single pair of panties I owned was stained. Before every period my abdomen bloated, blowing up to the point it was difficult to button even my most generously-cut skirts and pants. Because I was flowing so frequently, I felt as though I had a watermelon inside me most of the time.

ABOUT HOW TO DEAL WITH FIBROIDS

Often, fibroids require no treatment other than monitoring via regular medical visits.

But when fibroids cause serious problems, non-surgical options are limited. Some types of drugs, called Gn-RH agonists (gonadotropin-releasing hormone) can shrink fibroids by turning off the estrogen supply. Several such products are on the market, including Lupron, which is given by monthly injection, and Synarel, a daily nasal spray. But the benefits are only temporary, because these are powerful drugs that can be taken for a only few months. Once treatment stops, fibroids may return to their original size and keep on growing.

Holistic practitioners may suggest dietary changes such as cutting down or eliminating meat, poultry and dairy products, which may contain estrogens used in animal feeds, and consuming more whole grains, beans, vegetables and fruits. Others recom-

---

mend lifestyle changes such as reducing stress, exercising regularly and engaging in meditation or relaxation exercises.

Historically, physicians recommended hysterectomy if the uterus enlarged to the size of a twelve-week pregnancy. Surgery was the answer even if a woman had no other symptoms. In recent years a "wait and see" or "try other alternatives" attitude has become more common.

Unfortunately, for severe fibroids, as well as other types of problematic female conditions, surgery remains the only permanent solution.

Generally the most common indicators for hysterectomy or other surgical procedures are:

1. Uncontrollable or prolonged bleeding.

2. Pressure on adjacent organs, such as the bladder or bowel.

3. Pain.

4. A rapid change in size and consistency of the fibroids.

Many of these factors occur in combination, giving rise to quality-of-life issues ranging from frequent interruption of sleep to urinary incontinence to disruption of normal routine.

WHO? ME? HYSTERECTOMY?

For a long time I continued to believe my symptoms were menopause-related. After all, I was the right age, and hot flashes had me opening and closing windows so fast people around me quit trying to keep up. Variations in bleeding and irregular periods were frequently described as

~ ~

precursors of the change, and after thirty-five years of monthly visits, I was ready! On one wonderful occasion, I actually skipped a period! "Yes," I rejoiced, "no more bleeding, and with menopause, the end of fibroids."

That was the case, so the literature and my gynecologist told me, because once my supply of estrogen ceased, the fibroids would shrink and go away. With menopause apparently on the horizon, I was determined to wait out the problem.

The bleeding continued.

During regular, bimonthly visits to the gynecologist I persistently asked, "How much is too much?" I wanted him to tell me how much bleeding was abnormal. If I was soaking a super tampon and a super pad within twenty to thirty minutes, was that too much?

He couldn't tell me. Or wouldn't. Other questions about my bleeding got similarly vague answers. (I found out several years later, through my own research, that normal blood loss during an entire period should be no more than a third of a cup.) During office visits, it seemed like he was running a stop watch, allotting me only a pre-specified amount of time before moving on to the next patient. I considered shopping for another gynecologist; however, even though my insurance coverage was through the largest health maintenance organization in Michigan, gynecologists were in short supply. Going outside the plan to look for medical care was impossible; the cost would not be covered by insurance and I certainly could not handle the bills on my own.

To be certain the source of my bleeding was not a malignancy, the doctor performed an endometrial biopsy, using instruments to take samples of tissue from inside my uterus. The procedure was uncomfortable, but not really painful. I had cramping and bled for a few days afterward, but that was it.

Negative, thank God. But I kept flowing.

By late 1991, it was clear something needed to be done.

The gynecologist mentioned, rather casually I thought, "You could have a hysterectomy."

My response was simple — No! Emphatically not! I could not take the time off work; there was nobody to support me; it was just not possible or necessary. I was also determined not to be taken advantage of by the insensitive, yank-it-out medical establishment. I absolutely refused.

Besides, I had found a possible alternative, a relatively new procedure called endometrial ablation, which was being hailed not only as a way to control symptoms like mine, but by some doctors as a means of ending the inconvenience of having periods at all.

ABOUT SURGICAL OPTIONS

Four types of surgery are commonly available to deal with fibroids.

Endometrial ablation *uses a laser or cauterizing tool to burn away the lining of the uterus to control bleeding. This procedure, which makes pregnancy impossible, is generally done on an outpatient basis and requires a few days rest.*

Hysteroscopy *is the insertion of a hysteroscope, a slender instrument that is introduced through the cervix and allows the physician to examine the inside of the uterus. It is used in combination with a resecto-*

~ ~

scope, a tiny wire loop or laser. Using the resecto-scope, fibroids that are in the uterus may be cut off and removed. Effective only with fibroids that are inside the uterine cavity, this method may be used in outpatient surgery and requires only a few days rest.

Hysterectomy is the removal of the uterus and all attendant fibroids, permanently ending menstrual periods and the possibility of pregnancy. Depending on the size and location of fibroids, the surgery can be done vaginally or abdominally. In a vaginal hysterec-tomy, the uterus is detached, often using a laser tool called a laparscope, which is inserted through a small incision in the abdomen. The uterus is then taken out through the vagina. Abdominal hysterectomy requires an incision into the body cavity through the abdominal wall. Either method requires up to six weeks for resumption of a normal schedule and longer to regain full stamina and strength.

Myomectomy is the removal of fibroids only, leaving the uterus in place with the possibility of later pregnancy. The procedure can be performed with the laparscope inserted into the abdomen through a small cut near the naval or through an abdominal incision. Although myomectomy was introduced nearly a century ago, it has only recently gained in popularity. The operation is technically trickier than hysterectomy because each fibroid must be separated from the uterine wall and detached from its blood supply. This can lead to increased risk of excessive bleeding. The surgery can also take considerably longer than a hysterectomy, from four to six hours. A hysterectomy typically is completed in an hour or so. Removal of fibroids through a myomectomy does not guarantee that new fibroids will not grow, especially among

~ ~

> *younger women. Further surgery may be required at some point. Recovery from a myomectomy performed using laparoscopy may require only a brief hospital stay and a week or so of rest. Abdominal myomectomy may entail six weeks or more of recuperation.*

SURGERY #1

I first read about endometrial ablation in the newspaper. I clipped the article and showed it to the gynecologist during my next checkup. "Yes," he responded," I do that procedure; the hospital is just getting set up for it."

Wasn't it his job to bring the possibility of endometrial ablation to me?

For whatever reason, he did not. Although unnerved by this seeming role reversal, I was so relieved to find a way other than hysterectomy to address my problem that I did not push the issue.

We scheduled the surgery for early 1992.

In preparation, the doctor prescribed a series of monthly injections using the Gn-RH hormone-altering drug called Lupron Depot. The purpose was to shrink the fibroids, thin the lining of the uterus and slow down bleeding, so that the ablation would be easier to perform and more effective.

I received the injection; then, as scheduled, a second. Whoa!

Hot flashes, even while I was churning out laps in the swimming pool. Night sweats that drenched my body and the bedclothes, then set my teeth chattering as I chilled down. Tears that pooled up at the slightest provocation.

~ ~

Minutes of staring at the computer screen in my office without being able to organize my thoughts enough to write a single word.

The pamphlet I had gotten before the first injection of Lupron mentioned possible premenstrual and menopausal-like side effects of the drug, but I was completely unprepared for sensations as powerful as these.

Scariest was the thick gloom that surrounded me. I felt as if I were trying to move through bottomless gelatin, separated by the viscous substance from the world around me; tired, dulled, unable to push myself through to the surface. For the first, and I sincerely hope the only time in my life, I believe I had some sense of what clinical depression may be like. My will, my body and my spirit were paralyzed. I was so separated from the sense of myself that I often saw a part of me perch overhead like a vulture, watching the rest of me trying to act normally.

I called the clinic and discussed my reactions with the nurse. "Hang in there," she told me. "It should get better. Besides, you need the drug for the surgery."

Then the gynecologist slipped on the ice and broke his wrist.

With the surgery postponed for at least ten weeks, I called the nurse back and informed her that I would not be taking any more injections, that I would rather bleed than be depressed. (It was three years later that I found out Lupron, which was developed to treat endometriosis, had not been approved by the Federal Drug Administration for the purpose I received it.) When I stopped the shots, the symptoms lifted. Except for the bleeding, of course.

The endometrial ablation finally took place in June 1992. My son drove me to the surgical facility first thing in

~ ~

the morning. I was prepped and went into the operating room around 11 o'clock, woke up in recovery at 2:30 p.m. and by 4:30 p.m. was on the way home. I experienced considerable cramping and bleeding for four or five days, and an anesthesia hangover for two or three. But mostly I was optimistic: I had had the surgery. My bleeding was finished, at last!

Exactly one month later my period started. So much for endometrial ablation.

THINGS DID GET BETTER — FOR A WHILE

Actually I did have what were, more or less, normal periods. They lasted longer than those of many women, but I had always experienced that pattern. The blood clots were pretty much gone, the cramps were better and I wasn't spotting constantly. Still, I was disappointed that my periods had not stopped completely, as I had anticipated. Oh, well.

I continued to see the gynecologist regularly, so he could monitor me through examination and ultrasounds. When I asked why I was still having periods, he told me that endometrial ablation was less successful with women who have large fibroids high in the uterus, which I did. He also said that ablation does not work as well for women whose uteruses were tipped back, which mine was. Wasn't he supposed to know these things and tell me before the procedure, I thought to myself.

Gradually, over the next year or so, my symptoms came back. Longer periods, more and larger blood clots, stronger cramps and spotting without warning. I got in the

~ ~ ~ ~ ~ ~ ~ ~ ~ ~ ~ ~ ~ ~ ~ ~ ~ ~ ~ ~

habit of stashing pads and plugs everywhere because I never knew when I would need them. In my purse, my desk drawer at work, my briefcase, my knitting bag, my car, my bike bag, my ski jacket, my glasses case, my suit jacket pockets and in my bra if I had nowhere else to carry them.

During the heaviest days of my period, I would cover the sheets underneath me with a towel before going to bed. I knew I would have to get up two or three times during the night to change my pad and tampon, but sometimes, when I was especially tired, I did not awaken until I had soaked through everything. Because I was bleeding so much, I was tired a lot. At least the towel stopped the blood before it soiled the sheets — most of the time, anyway. More than once I turned over, off the towel, and was faced the next morning with having to wash not only the sheets but the mattress pad. Occasionally, the blood was so heavy it went through towel, sheets and mattress pad to the mattress itself.

Getting to work was another challenge. With a thirty-mile commute ahead of me, I learned to change everything just before I left the house. By the time I got to the office, after forty-five minutes in rush hour traffic, my first stop was always the ladies room, to change the super pad and tampon that had become heavy with clinging clots and discharged blood.

Worst of all was the gushing, which often happened when I stood up or moved suddenly. I am sure my face must have paled as the rush of hot blood burst from me. I know I muttered, "Oh, God, not again," hurrying to the bathroom to determine just how bad it was this time.

The intensity of my periods was setting off other problems, too. After several particularly heavy days of flow, my skin actually became raw and irritated from the constant chaffing of tampons and napkins. The internal pressure from my distended uterus on my bladder made me urinate frequently, and with great urgency. Constipation was another problem, no matter how much water I consumed.

Despite regular showers and careful personal hygiene, I felt like everyone knew when I was bleeding because of the faint odor I was convinced surrounded me. With the quick build-up of blood, and the constant changing of tampons and napkins, I felt, to use an old-fashioned term, "unclean."

"This Thing," as I began to think of it, took on an identity of its own. Rather than being an occasional, albeit essential part of a woman's life rhythms, my periods became a preoccupation. I was either about to start or was already bleeding, all the time. Premenstrual syndrome was my constant companion. My breasts were often swollen and tender, making me leery of a snuggling grandson with sharp elbows. Sex, too, was sometimes uncomfortable. My enlarged cervix was tender; contact could make me grimace with pain.

Despite all of this I valiantly adhered to my normal schedule, refusing to let my female problems curtail my activities or dictate how I ran my life. But several close women friends listened and watched and remarked that This Thing was taking more and more out of me as the months went by.

In fact, This Thing was making me crazy. The start of another period sent me into instant bitchiness and growling depression. I felt depleted and pale and irritable. "Damn, I just did this!" was my constant refrain.

Yet, I still hoped for menopause. My gynecologist assured me on every visit that I would get there very soon. I wanted so very much for him to be right.

Meanwhile, I kept on bleeding.

WHAT WAS IMPORTANT

As I contemplated hysterectomy, a number of issues influenced my thinking. Combining my analysis with the insights of other women, I offer what is, I hope, helpful advice at the end of each chapter.

1. Gather as much information as possible, from as many sources as possible. Even though the data is often contradictory, I wanted to know as much as I could.
2. Get educated about the female reproductive system, how it works, what kinds of problems can develop and what sorts of symptoms various conditions may cause. Knowing my own medical history was essential to understanding when things were not right.
3. Check on alternatives to hysterectomy, including less radical surgical procedures such as endometrial ablation, and possible drug therapies. Holistic remedies are available, too. In some cases, they might bring relief.
4. Get involved in your treatment. I found I had to ask if I wanted to get information from my physician. I even suggested my own treatments.

~ ~

Getting an adequate response was another matter.

5. Recognize that being your own advocate is not easy. As a layperson, it was difficult for me to keep up with developments in gynecology. I was even less sure how the doctor would respond to my suggestions.

6. See the doctor regularly. That was the only way I could ensure monitoring of my symptoms and keep even more serious medical conditions ruled out.

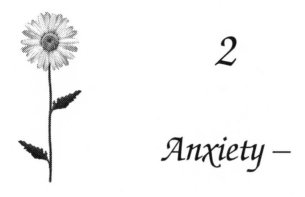

2

Anxiety –

Making A Decision

~ ~ ~ ~ ~ ~ ~ ~ ~ ~ ~ ~ ~ ~ ~ ~ ~ ~ ~ ~

The announcement seemed innocuous enough at the time. The company I work for had decided to switch to a different health insurance system. Since the new plan involved different providers, that meant switching doctors and clinic. A minor inconvenience.

Little did I know that the memo announcing the change was the first of several events that were about to coalesce. An accumulation of factors, coupled with my medical history, were finally about to push me into choosing to have a hysterectomy.

~ ~

WHAT TIPPED THE BALANCE

Knowing I had to find a new gynecologist when we changed health plans, I asked my friend Ann for her recommendation. The physician she had been seeing for several years was on our list of approved doctors, so I scheduled an appointment. (Freedom of choice regarding health care comes with a lot more strings attached than many of us may like to admit. The stark facts were, if I wanted full coverage of my medical expenses, my freedom to select a gynecologist existed within the confines of our company-sponsored managed care network. I was lucky; I finally found a gynecologist who was really good.)

I knew immediately that Dr. Meta Finn was someone I could relate to. First of all, she is a woman (which is not to say that male gynecologists may not be caring, compassionate, thorough and skillful). Fortyish, she was in my general age range. We could talk easily. She was willing to take time to listen and answer my questions. And during our first visit, when the topic turned to sports and exercise, she described her dream vacation — cross country skiing at Yellowstone. All right! I did not know it at the time, but the first of those final factors had just dropped into place.

A pelvic exam revealed my enlarged uterus. "Well, it's certainly big," she remarked. I explained my fervent wish to avoid hysterectomy, as well as my ongoing fibroid saga. To establish a baseline and get a better feel for the extent of my problem, she sent me for an ultrasound.

A week or so later I got a call from Dr. Finn at my office. In addition to the enlarged uterus and extensive fibroids throughout the organ, the ultrasound revealed an

~ ~

ovarian cyst. She explained that many women develop periodic cysts that simply go away as their cycles progress. She also indicated that a cyst that did not go away could indicate a much more serious problem — like a malignancy. She asked me if I was having any special pain or pressure. No. "Get another ultrasound," she said, "in six weeks. If the cyst is not gone, we'll have to evaluate what to do next."

That scared me. Despite my long-standing menstrual problems, this was the first indication that something more problematic could be happening inside me. I forgot to ask which ovary the cyst was on, but somehow I sensed it was the left one. That was later confirmed.

The cyst was the second of the factors that pushed me over the surgery brink.

Then my boyfriend Kal and I went up north to ski for the weekend, which was the occasion of my blood-in-the-snow episode (described in Chapter One). The period that precipitated that incident lasted for four weeks, not as a steady flow the entire time, but with heavy episodes connected with continual spotting. Despite having extended periods before, this was the longest one ever. Factor number three was in place.

I began thinking more seriously about having surgery — enough to make another appointment with Dr. Finn to talk about the possibility. Of course, she was extremely busy and it was several weeks before I could get in.

Meanwhile, investigating the whole subject of hysterectomy became a high priority, since I was now very personally involved.

NO WONDER WE'RE CONFUSED

My search for concrete answers yielded a lot more frustration than satisfaction. The aggravating truth was that rational, informed, objective discussion of the circumstances that might lead a woman to a hysterectomy, or to decide against it, was hard to come by.

Even attempting to educate myself was a challenge. Much of the data was contained in scientific journals that may not be available to the average woman and was difficult to understand and interpret, if she were to find them. Articles in the popular press were sometimes helpful, but just as often written to advocate a specific point of view.

According to several sources, the root cause of this lack of information, and the widespread uncertainty regarding the appropriateness of the surgery, can be traced, at least in part, to this astounding circumstance:

No long-term, randomized, controlled clinical trial has ever been conducted to determine the appropriate use of hysterectomy!

Similarly, no controlled clinical study has analyzed hysterectomy's long-term effects!

In practical terms that means professionals, laypeople, activists, writers and others have a variety of opinions, often contradictory, on the subject.

A sampling:

- "Hysterectomy is highly effective in relieving the symptoms associated with fibroid tumors, abnormal bleeding and chronic pelvic pain." ("Hysterectomy And Its Alternatives," *HealthFacts,* May 1994)

~ ~

- "Hysterectomy should not be the first line of defense against fibroids. In fact, if a doctor tells you that you must have your uterus removed and doesn't offer other options, find another doctor." (Christmas, et al. *Essence*, January 1994)
- "When fibroids do cause problems, surgery is the only workable treatment." (Dranov, *American Health,* September 1993)
- "More than 99 percent of fibroid tumors of the uterus are benign, and most require no treatment." (Dranov, *Good Housekeeping,* June 1992)
- "It is difficult to reconcile the prevalence of new or unresolved symptoms following hysterectomy and the generally high levels of satisfaction with it." (Demerstein, et al. *Hysterectomy, New Options And Advances)*
- "As time passed after hysterectomy, women became increasingly dissatisfied." (Cutler, *Hysterectomy; Before And After)*
- "One day I realized that I was living my life like an invalid: making cautious choices, avoiding certain places, grabbing afternoon naps because I was always exhausted. Worse, this uterus, which I was protecting so carefully, was draining my spirit, and life had lost its spontaneity. Finally I decided to take the doctors' advice [and have a hysterectomy].... Today, I feel 100 percent better. There were no complications, no side-effects, no emotional breakdowns." (Christmas, et al. *Essence*, January 1994)

~ ~

- "[Following surgery] ... she suffered from symptoms of estrogen deprivation. Her skin became like parchment. She was often depressed, extremely fatigued, had difficulty sleeping. Cellular changes occurred on the surface of her eyes.... Incapacitating bone and joint pain forced her into arm and leg braces within a year after surgery.... She experienced short-term memory loss.... She lost the intense maternal feelings she once had had for her children.... And she lost the sexual desire she had for her husband." (Rothberg, *Woman's Newspaper,* 1985)
- "Surveys consistently show that most women who have hysterectomies are pleased with the results." (Grimes, *The Lancet,* December 1994)
- "Hysterectomy can also bring about unwelcome sexual changes. Since the uterus plays a key role in orgasm, sex may become less pleasurable." (Dranov, *American Health,* September 1993)
- "Women who were orgasmic and sexually fulfilled before surgery usually resumed activities successfully four to six weeks after hysterectomy." (Strausz, *You Don't Need A Hysterectomy)*

And on and on and on. The more I looked, the more convinced I became that every possible point of view on the matter of hysterectomy was supported by some source or another.

Consider these book titles, for example, and the alternatives to hysterectomy proposed by the authors:

~ ~

No More Hysterectomies, by Dr. Vicki Hufnagel, who ascribes a possible loss of strength, vitality and self-esteem to absence of the uterus and menstruation, advised women with difficult female problems to consider a technique of her own design called Female Reconstructive Surgery. Dr. Stanley West, in *The Hysterectomy Hoax,* declares that a hysterectomy may do more harm than good, and goes on to suggest myomectomy, the piecemeal removal of fibroids, as the preferable surgery. When I read the title *You Don't Need A Hysterectomy* by Ivan Strausz, MD, I felt like a victim for even entertaining the notion that a hysterectomy might be advisable for me. (Despite the title, Dr. Strausz's book turned out to be an informed and rational account of the conditions that might lead to hysterectomy with a thorough discussion of other treatment possibilities.)

Finally, I found that five words pretty much summarized the state of thinking relative to this surgery:

"Hysterectomy lends itself to ambiguity." ("Hysterectomy And Its Alternatives," *Consumer Reports,* September 1990)

I had certainly found that out. Discovering that somebody else had reached the same conclusion did make me feel a bit better; at least I was not the only person who was confused.

The article went on to explain the source of the confusion.

"Apart from its use in some life-threatening diseases … it's done to improve the quality, rather than the length, of a woman's life…. In this often-gray area, hysterectomy may well be the most obvious treatment but not necessarily the best one for a given individual. The nature and severity of a problem, menopausal status and other factors affect the options a woman has for avoiding hysterectomy. And her motivation for avoiding it, whether for childbearing or for other reasons, can play an important role. Some alternatives to hysterectomy are no easier, safer or less painful than hysterectomy itself."

As a reasonably well-read person, especially in matters relating to my health, I was well aware of some of the alternatives, including the introduction in the past decade of lasers, hormones, drugs, alternative surgeries and holistic therapies that might preserve the uterus and treat female disorders in ways other than hysterectomy. I had even experienced several for myself. But beyond what point did hysterectomy become a consideration? And how did loss of the uterus affect other aspects of a woman's health? I could find few guidelines and even less agreement, no matter how many sources I consulted.

At the very least, in the words of Steven J. Bernstein, assistant professor of internal medicine at the University of Michigan School of Medicine, "There is very little an uninformed consumer can do to distinguish between an appropriate hysterectomy and an inappropriate one."(cited in "Hysterectomy Hesitation," *Harvard Health Letter,* December 1993)

Great.

Here I was, a woman trying to make a tough decision that would affect every aspect of the rest of my life. And the sad truth was, "You're on your own, lady!"

That made me angry. Why should that be?

Why, with a surgery as widespread as hysterectomy, had the most fundamental research never been conducted?

~ ~

Why didn't we know, beyond the obvious, how removal of the uterus affected women physically, sexually, emotionally and psychologically?

Where — in an era characterized by such feats as orbiting the planet, storing billions of bits of data on a fingernail-sized computer chip and tracing genetic characteristics to a single strand of DNA — where were the truly effective alternative treatments that would make hysterectomy unnecessary?

And why don't we have a more complete understanding of the role of the uterus and its contributions, beyond housing babies, to a woman's overall health and well-being?

I suspect the answers lie, to some extent at least, in the generalized neglect of women's health issues — like the fact that studies of factors contributing to heart disease have historically been conducted only with male subjects, even though coronary artery disease is the number one cause of death for women. In fact, women arriving at a hospital complaining of chest pains are less likely to be tested for a heart attack than men.

Cognizant though I was of all that, my frustration and anger were of little practical value in resolving my immediate, and ongoing, problem. I was still bleeding, a lot more than I thought was normal; but I could find no detailed discussion of that phenomenon either. The books and articles and pamphlets all mentioned "heavy" or "abnormal" bleeding, usually in the same sentence as "fibroids," along with endometriosis, adenomyosis, endometrial hyperplasia, pelvic relaxation, severe pelvic pain, pelvic inflammatory disease and, of course, cancer, as conditions that might lead to hysterectomy. But at what

~ ~

point did normal become excessive? How heavy was heavy?

And what about a discussion of the effect of bleeding in the overall context of a woman's life? How and why does heavy, frequent bleeding compromise lifestyle? Does it have to? Are there ways to resolve such issues other than the obvious, which was hysterectomy? That was precisely my dilemma.

At one point, I would have given my kingdom for a single, clear, concise, rational presentation of all the possibilities and alternatives available to me, coupled with a discussion of the advantages and drawbacks of each one.

Instead, I turned up a couple of facts about the surgery that reinforced my feeling that this was not a decision to be taken lightly. One woman in ten requires a blood transfusion during the operation; there is a complication rate of 5 percent to 20 percent (some sources claim rates of nearly 50 percent), although most complications are deemed to be not long-term or serious (also vigorously disputed in various writings); and people do die, at a rate of two per 1,000 operations for women between the ages of 45 and 65, or 600 a year. I also learned that death rates are higher among African-American women, as is the percentage of black women who have the surgery.

Another interesting finding I uncovered is that women who have the surgery tend to be well-insured. One study, conducted by the RAND Corporation (Bernstein et al, *Journal of the American Medical Association* May 12, 1993), in exploring the ongoing abuse-of-hysterectomy issue, set out to determine if various kinds of health plans gave physicians a financial incentive to perform these surgeries. Specifically, the study looked at whether the tradi-

~ ~

tional fee-for-service medical care system produced more hysterectomies than pre-paid medical groups where physicians were on salaries, and whether hysterectomies, when they were performed, had been done only after other therapies had been tried.

Underlying the methodology was the hypothesis that doctors in the salaried group might withhold care to save money, while those in the fee-for-service category could be recommending surgery for the opposite reason. What the study concluded was that the rate of what they deemed "inappropriate hysterectomy" was the same for both groups. An example of what this group called "inappropriate hysterectomy" was one done for a fibroid tumor smaller in size than a twelve-week fetus, with mild bleeding and no pain or discomfort in a women over age 40.

An example of an "uncertain indication," according to this research, was hysterectomy done for mild abnormal uterine bleeding. I felt my bleeding was beyond mild, but with no standards to go by, I was not sure. Persistent bleeding between periods was another example of questionable justifications. I did have this, although according to that study, this might not be sufficient cause to consider hysterectomy. Two other indications included being treated with one course of hormonal therapy (I had had Lupron and could not tolerate it), and one diagnostic evaluation of the uterine lining (I had had at least two, an endometrial biopsy and an analysis of the tissue following my endometrial ablation).

So, I asked myself, based on my symptoms, was I or was I not an appropriate candidate for hysterectomy?

~ ~

How, in the face of all the controversy and lack of research and dissension and dearth of information, was I supposed to make an informed decision about *me?*

Where I looked for clarity, I found contradiction. In place of answers, I formulated more questions. Beneath the skin of the competent, assured, decisive woman I believed myself to be, was a scared and confused little girl who wanted somebody else to tell her what to do.

ABOUT OTHER FEMALE PROBLEMS

In addition to fibroids, women may suffer from several other conditions that could indicate hysterectomy.

Endometriosis *is the abnormal growth of tissue that looks and acts like the endometrium, the lining of the uterus, in areas other than inside the organ. Little is known about why some women develop endometriosis, although it may be genetically influenced.*

The condition occurs only among menstruating women when normal endometrial tissue backs up with menstrual blood through the fallopian tubes. The misplaced tissue then implants and grows in other areas of the abdomen, such as the ovaries, tubes, outer surface of the uterus, bowel and similar pelvic structures. At the end of the monthly menstrual cycle, when hormones signal a period, endometrial tissue growing outside the uterus breaks up and is shed at the same time the normal lining of the uterus is discharged. Unlike menstrual fluid from the uterus, which flows freely out of the body, blood from abnormal tissue has no place to go. The body responds by surrounding the menstrual-type bleeding with inflam-

mation or by trying to absorb the blood back into the circulatory system. At the time normal menstrual bleeding ends, scar tissue forms around the infected areas, setting off a repeated cycle of bleeding and scarring that may cause severe pain or adhesions (abnormal tissue that binds organs together).

Infertility is a common complaint related to endometriosis. Pain during intercourse may also occur.

Treatment for endometriosis includes hormonal therapy, with drugs given to temporarily alter normal female patterns and thus slow the growth of the misplaced tissue. Conservative surgery, often using laparoscopy, may remove spots of endometriosis from their abnormal locations. In severe cases, hysterectomy may be required.

Pelvic adhesions involve an irritation of the peritoneum, the tissue that lines the inside of the abdomen, causing scarring or adhesions. The adhesions bind the surfaces of affected organs together, causing pain. The irritations may be produced by endometriosis, infection or injury, and most commonly affect the back surface of the uterus, the tubes and ovaries, as well as the intestines.

Pelvic relaxation and **uterine prolapse** occurs when ligaments supporting the pelvic organs weaken due to inadequate development or childbearing and birth. The lack of support can cause the organs to bulge or otherwise rearrange in the abdominal cavity. If the uterus drops into the vagina or even outside the body, the condition is referred to as uterine prolapse. Pelvic relaxation may cause difficulty in controlling urine, as well as a sensation of pressure in the abdominal area.

~ ~

Cancer, malignant tumors in the uterus, cervix or ovaries, can cause abnormal bleeding if in the uterus, or no symptoms at all if in the ovaries. Immediate surgical removal of all female reproductive organs is indicated, with further treatment often required.

Other conditions that can lead to hysterectomy include adenomyosis, chronic pelvic pain, pelvic inflammatory disease and endometrial hyperplasia.

Adenomyosis, the benign invasion of the endometrium into the myometrium, generally causes symptoms only late in a woman's reproductive years. Heavy, prolonged bleeding and intermenstrual bleeding are the most common; nonspecific pelvic pain and bladder and rectal pressure can also occur. The uterus may be enlarged and misshapen; fibroidnomas are frequently present as well. In severe cases, hysterectomy may be indicated.

Endometrial hyperplasia, which may be considered a precancerous condition, occurs when the lining of the uterus is incompletely and irregularly discharged during the monthly period. Bleeding becomes irregular, prolonged and sometimes profuse. Treatment can be complicated and must be individualized based on age, history, reproductive desires and severity of bleeding. A dilation and curettage (D and C), and various drug therapies, including oral contraceptives, may provide relief, although once treatment is discontinued new episodes can occur. Periodic endometrial biopsies are indicated to monitor development of malignancy. Hysterectomy provides the only permanent solution.

~ ~

MORE INQUIRY

Meanwhile, I continued to seek other information that might inform my choice.

I checked out my company's medical leave policy. Twenty-one days at full pay, after taking a first week at no pay or using vacation to cover the time. A total of 26 days at full pay; not exceptionally generous, but probably enough to cover the basic recovery period I would need. Fortunately, I felt secure enough in my contribution to the company to believe I would have a job upon recovery (real job security being a myth). Also, federal law requires reinstatement after a disability leave of absence.

Although I would have liked a longer paid medical leave, I knew I was fortunate to have what I did. Many women who suffer problems that might indicate hysterectomy do not have steady employment or sufficient income, medical insurance or the other resources that allowed me to eliminate those considerations from my decision-making. In that regard I was lucky.

Family considerations were also a factor. I was long past the point of wanting to have more children, so that was not an issue I had to consider. I also knew that my children, at 28 and 22, were old enough to carry on in the unlikely event I were to die or be incapacitated. Again, I knew I was fortunate and that many women in my situation could not dismiss such matters so easily.

Emotional support was another area in which I was lucky. My relationship with Kal was long-term and strong. I knew he would stand by me, no matter what I should decide.

~ ~

In gathering necessary information, I did a lot of talking to a lot of people.

I discussed hysterectomy with anyone I could find who had had one. Colleagues, coworkers, friends — I asked these women whether or not having a hysterectomy was the right decision. To a one, they answered with a resounding "yes!", adding affirmations like "You'll wonder afterward why you waited so long." Naturally I was heartened by their confirmations, but at the same time, I was confused.

On the one hand, I was reading reams of data that said hysterectomy was, if not downright unnecessary, at least widely abused; that having the surgery would cause dreadful consequences, perhaps damaging me permanently and undoubtedly ruining my sex life. Yet, right here in front of me were women I knew and liked and trusted, telling me a very different story. They were saying they felt better after having a hysterectomy than they had felt in years, that they had suffered no long-term negative effects, even sexually. Several said the same thing in answer to my anxious questions: "Having a hysterectomy was the best thing I ever did for myself."

Who was I supposed to believe?

Surely my mother was a reliable source. She was 52 when she underwent her hysterectomy. She, too, suffered from fibroids, which had caused her heavy, frequent bleeding for years. She said, "It had gotten to the point I was so anemic I couldn't walk up the stairs in the house without the top of my head throbbing from the exertion. The doctor told me I had fibroids, at least two large ones, the size of an orange and a grapefruit. But he didn't really recommend a hysterectomy, and I thought I'd go into menopause and the bleeding would stop." Like mother, like daughter.

~ ~

My mom's moment of truth came when she stood up to sing the final hymn at the end of a church service. Her description of what happened is graphic : "The bottom fell out. I wasn't wearing a pad or anything because I'd finished a period several days before and thought I didn't need protection. I started hemorrhaging. I quickly sat down and waited until everyone left the church. Another lady nearby saw what had happened and came to sit with me. Your dad went to the rest room and brought back a bunch of paper towels. I left a trail of blood all the way to the car. When we got home, your dad got a towel, but I still dripped blood everywhere. The next day I went to the doctor and a week later I had a hysterectomy."

She also told me, which I had not known previously, that her mother had experienced bleeding problems. My grandma had to keep a chamber pot by her bed because she was unable to get to the bathroom without bleeding all over the floor. Still, Grandma never had a hysterectomy. She eventually stopped bleeding with menopause, and went on to live to the robust age of 86 before quietly slipping away one morning at home in her bed. If she had made it without surgery, why couldn't I?

Continuing the family connection, I grilled my sister, who is a physician and board-certified internist, for her medical and personal advice. The genetic component of female problems was certainly evident in our case, although my sister's primary problem was endometriosis rather than fibroids. Eventually she had laser surgery to remove scar tissue that was causing severe abdominal pain. "I'm not very optimistic about the future of my uterus," she once told me. The source of her dilemma, in addition to a demanding career, a husband and two young sons, was the desire to have another child.

I discussed the matter, pro and con, with Kal, especially my fears that such a momentous change in my physiology might affect our relationship. He reassured me that he would love me, even without a uterus. Not wanting to risk a self-fulfilling prophecy, I let the matter rest, without telling him how deeply concerned I really was.

Meanwhile, I found it increasingly difficult to avoid waking up during the night to worry. I was haunted by one particular horror story, about a woman whose husband dropped her and her suitcase at the door of the hospital when she went in for a hysterectomy. He did deign to pick her up after the surgery, but filed for divorce soon after that.

My fears about the affect of a hysterectomy were no doubt exacerbated by the fact I was a single woman. Although Kal and I were a committed couple, we were not married, and I was all too familiar with the fragility of relationships between men and women. Like most single women, I had been hurt by men who walked away at the first sign of adversity, or who terminated a relationship when they sensed themselves getting too close. I knew Kal was not like that, that he viewed the possibility of my having a hysterectomy as something that was necessary and that we would deal with it and move on. Still, there was a fear, born of past disappointments, that he would choose not to be bothered. And what would happen if for some awful reason we were no longer together? Would I be desirable to other men? Even more nagging, would I still feel desire? I really was not sure.

DECISION TIME? NOT QUITE

Finally, after all my dithering and talking and worrying, the day came for my long-awaited appointment with Dr. Finn came. The day of decision, when I would finally come to a resolution to this vexing issue. According to Kal, I had already made up my mind and was just waiting for confirmation from my doctor that surgery was the right thing to do.

Two hours before I was due at the doctor's, the phone rang at my office.

"You have an appointment at noon with Dr. Finn?"

"Yes."

"This isn't an emergency, correct?"

"Well, no, not really, but I have some urgent concerns."

"You're basically coming in to talk, right?"

I said I guessed so.

"Dr. Finn is canceling — she is not feeling well...."

I did not hear another word, especially when I found out I could not get another appointment for a week.

I lost it! I absolutely fell apart! I slammed down the phone, yelling, with numerous expletives. "I don't believe it! They can't do this to me!" I ran from my office to the rest room, and struggled for some minutes to stop shouting and swearing and regain a semblance of control. I was absolutely convinced mine was the only appointment canceled. I believed my case was not considered important; that the doctor, for whatever reason, blew me off. That was not true, of course. When I talked to Dr. Finn by phone a couple of days later, she had such severe laryngitis that she could barely whisper. But in my agitated mental state I was

~ ~

convinced that the cancellation of my appointment was personal, that "they" dumped me for some malicious reason.

Somehow I made it through the rest of the day at the office. I was in the midst of an extensive and extremely demanding project that had been fraught with setbacks and revisions, and it did nothing to improve my mental state.

All the way home I cried hysterically, tears running onto my coat. I drove around my neighborhood for two hours, sobbing and yelling. "They can't do this to me! Why did they do this to me? Why wasn't I important? Why did they dump me?" My daughter and grandsons were staying with me at the time and I could not go home and face them, not when I was so frantic.

Finally, about 8:30 p.m., I recognized I out of control. I stopped at a phone booth and called Kal. I shivered — it was a blustery, snowy, Michigan March night — as I cried into the receiver. I explained the cancellation, demanding to know why the doctor had dismissed me. Kal was worried, as was my daughter, who had called him several times.

Did I want him to come and get me? No, I thought I could make it to his house on my own. Would he call my daughter and tell her I was okay and on the way to his place? Yes, he'd be glad to. I started the long drive to his home, thirty miles across town. His calmness on the phone and his reasonable approach to my distress helped settle me down enough to get there safely. He was waiting for me with a hot cup of coffee and warm, sympathetic arms.

In thinking later about this episode, I was amazed at the ferocity of my reaction to the cancellation. After all, the situation was straightforward: the doctor was ill, and as a result was forced to postpone her appointments. That should

~ ~

have been that; disappointing perhaps, but nothing more. Instead, I flew into an emotional explosion completely out of character for me. Normally, I was a level-headed problem-solver; I routinely made major decisions as part of my job and my life. But this was different. The question of having a hysterectomy was one that carried consequences, many of which were ambiguous, that would be with me the rest of my life.

The only explanation I have for my hysteria on this day is that I was so tightly wound and emotionally invested in resolving this long-standing issue that the forced delay sent me over the edge. Did I overreact to the postponement? Absolutely! But my tirade was, I believe, symptomatic of my level of distress.

Throughout this entire period, the tension of making a decision, while still faced with the necessity of carrying on with normal living, pushed me into an elevated state of emotionalism the likes of which I had experienced few times before in my life. I was bitchy, short-tempered, impatient and easily frustrated. Minor everyday hassles, like freeway slowdowns and long supermarket lines, could send me into a fury. I was preoccupied and psychologically fragile, getting misty-eyed over silly television commercials, stumbling over curbs because I was not paying attention, forgetful of everything except my dilemma.

GETTING ANSWERS

The week between the cancellation and my rescheduled appointment went by quickly, and I was able to use the time to get some necessary things done. I had another ultrasound, I collected my records from the previous gynecolo-

~ ~

gist and I read and reread an article on hysterectomy that appeared, fortuitously, in the *Detroit Free Press* right at that time. This balanced, intelligent treatment of hysterectomy was just what I needed — a concise consideration of common female problems and a listing of some of the various options available, without making judgments either way. The article urged women to ask questions, explore alternatives and become advocates in the crucial decisions affecting their life and health. I found the piece extremely helpful, reassuring me that I was going about making my decision in the right way.

When it was finally time for my new appointment, I arrived at Dr. Finn's office, armed with a page-long list of questions. I was determined to get an idea of what I was facing, if I did decide to go ahead.

First, we reviewed my records. The new ultrasound revealed that, in comparison to the studies ordered by my previous doctor, my fibroids were definitely on the move. And there was not just one; my entire uterus was involved. Dr. Finn estimated I was four months pregnant, except the only thing I was pregnant with was misplaced uterine tissue. The ovarian cyst was not visible, although, as we found out during the actual surgery, it was still there.

With that information in mind, I handed Dr. Finn one copy of my list of questions, and I kept the other. We dug in.

Dr. Finn, to her credit and my gratitude, was willing to spend the time I needed answering my inquiries.

For example:

Q: What were the medical indications supporting my having this surgery?

~ ~

A: Four-week-long periods, anemia, an enlarged uterus, growing fibroids, cramps, heavy bleeding, clotting.

Q: Were there alternatives to hysterectomy?

A: Endometrial ablation was one, but I had already tried that. D and C was another, but the results would likely be the same as with the ablation — relief for a while, then the fibroids could grow again and the bleeding escalate.

Q: What kind of surgical technique were we talking about? Could laparoscopy and a vaginal procedure be used to avoid an abdominal incision?

A: In my case, no, because my uterus was too large and the fibroid involvement too extensive. (Dr. Finn indicated that some physicians were willing to go in and shave down a large uterus to remove it piece by piece; she felt such a procedure put the patient under anesthesia for too long — 4 or 5 hours — creating more risk than an incision would, and might leave fibroids outside the uterus behind.)

Q: What about the ovaries? What were the chances that the cyst was malignant? Should I have them taken out?

A: There was no way to gauge the condition of the cyst without looking at it and taking tissue samples. Having the ovaries out was my decision; I could think about it, up until the day of surgery, if necessary. If I did decide to have the ovaries removed, I would go on synthetic hormones immediately to head off instantaneous menopause.

~ ~

Q: Should I have a bladder suspension as part of the surgery?

A: She had not considered that, and a urologist would have to make the determination. She could recommend two that she trusted and try to set up an immediate appointment for me.

Q: How long would I be in the hospital?

A: Three to four days, depending on my insurance coverage.

Q: How long after surgery would I bleed and how much?

A: Three to four weeks, although after the first few days the discharge should be light and brownish in color.

Q: How long was the recovery period and what should I expect to feel and do during that time?

A: Six weeks before returning to work and resuming a more or less normal schedule. I could expect to be extremely fatigued, even after the more overt symptoms, such as pain, had subsided.

Q: How soon could I exercise? Drive? Have sex?

A: Four to six weeks to exercise. Two to three to drive. Six before having sex.

Q: Would sex be affected? Should I be concerned about having a good sexual relationship with a good man and not wanting to mess that up?

A: Ninety percent of sex drive is between the ears, not the legs. Once I was healed, there was no reason why my sex life should be diminished. Of course, hormone therapy adjustment is important to a woman if her ovaries have been taken.

Too low a dosage could affect the libido. Also,
some women are more sensitive in the cervical
area than others. If I was one of those, it was
possible that my sexual sensations could be
affected.

Q: How soon could we schedule the surgery? I had
to be up and more or less normal by May 14,
when my son was to be best man at his best
friend's wedding.

A: That depended on the hospital and availability of
the urologist.

I had a choice of hospitals, since Dr. Finn was on staff
at two in the area — a large, urban medical center and a
smaller neighborhood facility. Although both had excellent
reputations, I indicated my preference for the latter. I had
already made inquiries in the neighborhood and knew the
smaller hospital provided thorough and attentive care.

We discussed the relative merits of myomectomy vs.
hysterectomy. Being aware of the role of the uterus in relationship to overall health and sexual pleasure, I wondered if
a myomectomy might be possible. In my case, a myomectomy would still require an abdominal incision, and the
extent of my fibroids made it unlikely all could be removed.
Since the recovery period was sometimes even longer for a
myomectomy than a hysterectomy, and I did not want to
have more children, doing it that way did not seem to make
much sense.

I also asked about sub-total hysterectomy – removing
the uterus while leaving the cervix in place. In many women
the cervix is responsive to sexual stimulation; by preserving
that part of the uterus, possible changes in sexual response
after hysterectomy may be lessened. I had read that only 1

~ ~

percent of surgeries done in the United States involve sub-
total hysterectomy. That percentage is much higher else-
where; in Sweden, for example, supracervical hysterectomies are as high as 21 percent. Dr. Finn responded that
one of the biggest reasons more sub-total procedures are not
done here has to do with insurance coverage; most companies will not cover this type of procedure, in part because
leaving the cervix leaves a potential site, however remote,
for the development of cancer at some later time.

Dr. Finn urged me to get another opinion, if that
would help me in making a decision. In essence I had
already done that, since she was the second gynecologist to
mention hysterectomy as a possible remedy to my long-
standing problems.

I recounted the struggles and confusion I had been
experiencing in determining whether a hysterectomy was
the right choice for me. "It's not easy," she confirmed.
"Your uterus is certainly an integral and important part of
you, and what happens there is connected to your entire
bodily system. We honestly don't know everything we
should about what happens when we remove it. Knowing
that, you have to take into account all you know about your
condition and your circumstances, and decide for yourself
how miserable you are and whether you can and want to
continue to live the way you are now."

Dr. Finn made an interesting observation as we
discussed the recovery period: She indicated that her hard-
driving, high-achieving patients sometimes had a rougher
recovery than calmer, more sedentary women. The difference seemed to be that the Type As had trouble slowing
down enough to let their bodies heal, while patients who
were more relaxed by nature and kept less demanding

schedules found it easier to relax. It was pretty obvious which category she felt I fell into.

REALITY CHECK

During the consultation, Dr. Finn handed me her hysterectomy surgical consent form. It was no nonsense, just like she was. The form said:

I am a candidate for hysterectomy; I agree to the surgery.

I know that the decision to have, or not to have a hysterectomy is entirely up to me.

I can decide NOT to have a hysterectomy.

A discussion of the procedure came next.

The procedure of hysterectomy, the removal of the uterus and cervix only, has been discussed with me, with its risks and side effects, recovery and disability post-op.

I understand that a hysterectomy is permanent and not reversible. I understand that by having my uterus removed I will no longer be able to get pregnant, bear children or have menstrual periods.

The next part, about risks, was almost enough to send me into a hasty retreat from the entire program.

I understand that there are risks and side effects to any surgery, which can range from minor to fatal:

- *I could have a reaction to, or an undesirable outcome from, anesthesia.*
- *I could lose more blood than expected and might require a blood transfusion. Although the need for transfusion is unpredictable, the risks of a*

~ ~

transfusion — possible reactions, hepatitis, HIV, etc., are known to me.

- *I could develop a serious infection, which might require longer hospitalization with antibiotics or other treatments or additional surgery.*
- *Because the abdominal cavity will be entered, there is the potential to accidentally injure any organ within the abdomen, such as the tubes and ovaries, the urinary bladder, the intestines, pelvic nerves, the ureters or blood vessels.*
- *Any such injury may require immediate or later surgery to correct.*
- *Serious blood clots could form in my legs or lungs from lying inactive after surgery. Pneumonia could develop for the same reason.*
- *A bladder or urinary infection could result from the catheter draining the bladder.*
- *If I have a general anesthesia, I may expect to have a sore or scratchy throat later.*
- *There could be blood collections called "hematomas," bruising or pain at the IV sites, the incision or places wherever blood has been drawn.*
- *I could have nausea, vomiting, pain, poor healing, hernia formation or scarring.*

I understand that it is impossible to list every possible undesirable effect, and in some cases, the condition for which the surgery is done is not always cured or improved and in some cases may even be made worse.

~ ~

There was some additional discussion covering such issues as hospitalization, recovery, pain relief and finally, smoking.

If I am a smoker, I understand that I should stop prior to surgery.

Fortunately, I was not, so I met that requirement easily.

Finally, there was a place for me to sign. She told me not to do so yet, until I had read the form thoroughly several times and found a witness to my signature.

Dr. Finn gave me a pamphlet to read, *Understanding Hysterectomy,* published by the American College of Obstetricians and Gynecologists. There I learned:

Although hysterectomy is considered major surgery, the surgical risk is one of the lowest of any major operation.

I asked what the term "major surgery" means in the medical lexicon. Dr. Finn described it as any procedure where there was a substantial risk of something going wrong. The pamphlet continued by spelling out those "somethings."

As with any major abdominal or pelvic opera-tion, serious complications, such as blood clots, severe infection, post-operative hemorrhage, bowel obstruction, injury to the urinary tract or even death, can occur.

Not very reassuring, but I wanted to be as fully aware as I could of what might befall me. The pamphlet concluded:

The risks and possible benefits of any opera-tion must be evaluated before surgery is advised.

In the final analysis, my thinking centered on the *benefits* side of the equation — no more periods that went on forever, no more heavy bleeding, no more cramps and blood clots and gushing, no more swollen abdomen, no more anemia, no more preoccupation with "This Thing."

I decided to go ahead, with Dr. Finn's assurance that I could still change my mind.

Then, of course, I was anxious to get it all over with — immediately. "That's pretty typical," my doctor told me. "Once women finally decide to have the surgery, they usually want to have it right now."

I left her office with a tentative surgery date and an appointment to see the urologist to discuss a possible bladder suspension.

Is It Always So Tough?

No. A number of the women with whom I talked while researching this book reported they came much more easily than I did to the decision to have a hysterectomy. Like Jody.

"I'd been hemorrhaging for three years. When I'd stand up, clots the size of tennis balls would come out. At one point I was on the golf course up north when I started gushing right through my clothes. In front of all those strange people. Then I had three Pap smears in a row that didn't look right and were progressively worse. At that point, my doctor said, 'What would you think about a hysterectomy?' and I said, 'Do it!' I never had a second thought. I was 38 years old. Of course, I've got five kids and there's no way in hell I'd ever have

~ ~

another one, so I didn't even have to think about that part of it."

Lynn, who is a physician, described her hysterectomy as "a very clinical decision. It needs to come out? Okay, let's do it tomorrow." Lynn's problem was a big fibroid mass — "so large I could feel it pressing inside of me when I got on the Nordic Trak" — complicated by widespread endometriosis and a large, blood-filled cyst on the left ovary. Despite all that, Lynn did not experience abnormal bleeding or pain, although the increasing size of the fibroid was pressuring her bladder. "Then my gynecologist got worried that the rapid growth of the fibroid indicated malignancy. My dad had just died and a good friend was dying of cancer right at that time, which made my condition really frightening until we got the results of the biopsy. That turned out to be negative, thank God, but then I just wanted to have it gone." Like Jody, Lynn was 38 at the time of her surgery. "The kid issue was never a problem for me, because I'm not going to have any. Later an old beau called up and said what a bummer it was not to be able to have any kids. But I didn't care about that."

Lea had constant bleeding and endometriosis, complicated by a low iron level. Although she had been taking iron for a year and half before surgery, at age 37 her body was not accepting the supplements.

"I had a D and C for the bleeding but that didn't help. Actually, I'd had problems with cramping ever since I was a kid, and I was really sick of it — the constant cramps, always feeling so weak, working full time on top of all that. I had two kids, and I knew I wasn't having any more because I'd already had a tubal ligation. So when my doctor

starting talking about hysterectomy, I just said,
'Schedule it, please!' I was so ready! My husband
said he'd never seen anybody so excited. I talked a
lot to my mother and sister, who'd both had
hysterectomies, and had done very well."

Helen was similarly emphatic. Like Lea, she had had
two children and a tubal ligation to prevent having any
more. At 47, she had two huge fibroids, causing typical
symptoms of heavy bleeding and cramping, which she and
her doctor had been monitoring for two years.

"He never would tell me, 'You have to have a
hysterectomy.' He said I had to tell him. So finally I
did. There's absolutely no question in my mind that
a hysterectomy was what I needed."

"The women in my family have a long history of
severe osteoporosis, which prompted my doctor to start me
on hormones as I got near to menopause," was how Mary's
story began. "But I also had fibroids, and the extra
hormones led to intermittent bleeding between my periods.
So I had a D and C to control the bleeding. But my uterus
was full of fibroids, which continued to grow even after I
stopped taking hormones. I finally decided to have a
hysterectomy while my uterus was still small enough that I
could have it removed vaginally. My insurance required a
second opinion, so I went to a male gynecologist and
explained that my doctor was planning a vaginal procedure.
He was so arrogant! He didn't even bother to examine me,
just said he'd insist on cutting me open so he could see
everything. Even though he made me mad, he scared me.
My regular doctor (a woman) talked to me at length,
though, and I felt better. We went ahead as planned."

~ ~

"These problems develop so gradually," said Alice, referring to the bleeding that accompanied her fibroids, "that we adjust our lives to accommodate them. Like a lot of other women, I just learned to cope. The truth is, we run out of alternatives very quickly. But after a while, the bleeding was controlling me; plus my bladder really started taking a beating. It was displaced because my uterus was so large. I finally had the hysterectomy when I had blown up to the size of a five-month pregnancy, and one of the fibroids looked suspicious — solid — which was very frightening. It took me two days after the pathology report came back to really believe it was negative."

Still, hysterectomy is not a matter to be undertaken lightly, as Donna's experience attests:

"I was 46, with excessive bleeding and pain on one side. And I was anemic; I'd come home from work and just lay on the couch, I was so tired. I finally decided I couldn't go on living that way, but I wasn't sure having a hysterectomy was the right thing to do. I made a list of all the positives and negatives, the pros and cons of the surgery, as best I could figure out. That wasn't easy, because there is so much conflicting information. I studied all the elements and weighed all the factors before I made my decision."

My conversations with these women and a number of others about how they arrived at the decision to have a hysterectomy brought out what appear to be some important, common themes.

First was that while the types of female problems varied, they were generally long-standing and, by the time of the surgery, getting worse. Many women described years of pain, bleeding, clotting, cramping, bloating, anemia and other symptoms. For the most part, they attempted to carry on with business as usual, or make subtle adjustments in their lives to cope. Typically, they came to surgery, as I did, as a last resort, when all else had failed. In many cases, they had tried alternative treatments, most often a D and C, or, as in my case, an endometrial ablation and drug therapy, without gaining significant relief.

Many women spoke of the physical drain their conditions caused them, and the compromises they had made in their lifestyles. "My bleeding and pain and weakness had become the focus of my existence," was how one woman put it. "It gets to the point it affects every single part of you, and that's not good."

Said another, "Because we're women, we're used to carrying on. So we take two aspirin and drag ourselves to work, no matter what. But there were days when I was so weak I could hardly think."

The issue of "carrying on" was important to many of us as we tried to cope with our physical symptoms. I know I went to great lengths not to let my bleeding curtail my activities (other than sex, when my periods got really bad). As a woman in business, working for a company and with clients who were predominantly male, I was especially anxious not to appear weak or in any way compromised by being a woman. I worked hard to conceal how I was feeling, even from those closest to me. I knew my ceaseless litany of symptoms must get tiresome — I was certainly bored with it, and I did not want to burden others with my problem.

Even Kal said later he did not realize how much I was being affected by my problems until he read this book. "Gee," he laughed. "People must wonder why I kept

~ ~

hanging out with this 'bloody' woman who was always running to the bathroom or wetting her pants." He added, more seriously, "I knew you were having problems, but you never let on you were in such bad shape."

The fact is, most of us with these kinds of female problems just get through them somehow, often staging award-caliber performances, until things get so bad we are forced to make another choice.

Putting the matter into perspective after her hysterectomy, another woman concluded, "You don't realize how bizarre what you're going through is until you're not doing it anymore." I certainly agree with that.

A second conclusion I came to after researching hysterectomy was the fact that no two sets of circumstances were precisely the same. One patient, who was a nurse, observed that there were at least as many different reasons for having a hysterectomy as there were types of apples. Of the women I talked to, several had fibroids, others had endometriosis, one had a prolapsed uterus, still another had chronic pelvic pain of unspecified origin, and in some instances, women exhibited various combinations of several conditions. There was one case of ovarian cancer, although a leaky appendix had led to the discovery of the malignancy, probably allowing detection early enough to save the woman's life. And in yet another instance, hysterectomy came as a by-product of primary surgery for urinary incontinence.

That so many different types of conditions can lead to hysterectomy contributes to the ambiguity and controversy that surround the surgery. The lack of clear-cut guidelines to indicate appropriateness leaves a woman in a difficult and troubling position, especially when so many variations,

~ ~

combinations and permutations of symptoms and conditions can end up in the operating room.

One of the few things women dealing with hysterectomy agreed on was the lack of good information.

"This was a fragile, emotional decision, even though I was convinced having a hysterectomy was the right choice for me," recalled Alice. "There were so many unknowns, about what I could expect to happen to me, during the surgery and as I recovered — sex, hormone replacement, how I'd feel, how to cope. I did find a book that was very helpful. It's been a year since my surgery, and I'm still referring to it to find out what's next."

With no clear description of "normal," it is even more difficult for women to gain understanding of their options. Lynn, the physician, put it succinctly: "Women need a discussion of choices, so we can know what we're deciding about."

Without a more formal and reasoned assessment, women turn, as I did, to their friends and relatives for information about hysterectomy.

"That helped fill up some of the dark holes for me," recalled Helen. "And I'm a nurse, a medical professional. I can't imagine what women do who lack the resources and contacts I had. We're finally talking openly about menopause and breast cancer. It's time to do the same for hysterectomy."

"I know I didn't ask enough questions, and didn't have enough information about hysterectomy, even though I was miserable beforehand," said Cheryl. Then she got to the real horror story. "But the woman in the bed next to me was much worse off. Her doctor never told her what hysterec-

~ ~

tomy does to women. I'm not sure she even knew she couldn't get pregnant anymore."

Which raises another of the crucial elements of a woman's decision about hysterectomy — the relationship with her physician.

"Implicit trust" was how several women described their feelings. In one case, despite a malpractice suit that had been settled against her doctor, a woman reported that she "liked and trusted him so much I knew he would do the right thing for me."

"It's so great as a woman of 51," said another of my confidants, "to finally find a doctor who doesn't make you embarrassed to ask absolutely any question you want."

But how does a woman know what questions to ask? "If you think of it, ask it," seems to be the rule to go by. "Be an advocate for your own health," as one woman said. "The more empowered you feel in making your decision, the better off you'll be," agreed another. "But I know we don't always know how to do that."

Compounding the problem are attitudes that do not always encourage women to do that. "Does the 'hyster' part of 'hysterectomy' stand for 'hysterical?'" questioned one candidate for the surgery, "because that's how one doctor made me feel."

Another reported encountering an "it will go away" attitude on the part of both doctors and insurance companies. She concluded, rather bitterly, "If men and insurance companies went through what we do every month, a lot of rules would be different."

Women who told me about unhappy experiences with hysterectomy did not report a high level of trust and confidence in their doctors, nor a feeling of having taken an

~ ~

active role in decision-making. "I was so young and naive," said a woman who nearly bled to death following a vaginal hysterectomy performed in 1971, when she was 32 years old. "In those days they just automatically did a hysterectomy for any kind of female problem. And I did have problems; I'd bleed for four weeks at a time and then skip the next six months. But I just blindly believed everything the doctor told me."

"I went into surgery crying and I came out crying," recalled a woman who was presented with a form consenting to the removal of her ovaries on the way to the operating room. "The doctor didn't even mention taking out my ovaries along with my uterus until it was too late for me to think about what I was doing. So I signed. The whole thing was so high-handed. And the doctor was a woman. Then, several months after the surgery, when I complained about being depressed and crying all the time, she told me to go see a psychiatrist. Her attitude clearly was, 'You had my surgery, so I'm done with you'."

As my experience and those of other women illustrate, the decision to have a hysterectomy ranks among the most monumental choices any woman will have to make during the course of her entire life. Lack of information, and the contradictory nature of so much of what does exist, means that we must make our choices in an atmosphere of swirling ambiguity and frustrating uncertainty.

The bottom line is, surgery is an irreversible step, and any woman deciding to undergo hysterectomy, and related procedures, must carefully weigh the risks and benefits in the context of her own life.

Ultimately, I had to rely on my own intuition, guided by the counsel of other women, my doctors and my reading, to arrive at the decision that I believed was right for me.

WHAT WAS IMPORTANT

My advice for women faced with the hysterectomy dilemma.

1. Find a gynecologist you like and can relate to. Dr. Finn was someone I could talk with; she was honest and straightforward, and she was willing to take time to answer my questions and address my fears. I had sufficient confidence in her professional skills to trust her, literally, with my life.

2. Check out the hospital you will be going to. The surgical hospital was also critical to my well-being, so I made a point of asking around about the facility where my doctor preferred to work. Good word-of-mouth in the community was especially important, because I figured people would certainly tell me if they felt their health or that of loved ones was compromised during a hospital stay.

3. Read everything you can find. To assure myself that the surgery was medically indicated, I studied all the material I could locate on my symptoms and ways to resolve them.

4. Do not believe everything you read. As I have detailed, much of the information is, at best, ambiguous, and frequently, downright contradictory.

5. Talk to other women about their decisions and their experiences. Real-world, personal histories were the best source of comfort and reassurance I could find.

6. Seek a second and even a third or fourth opinion about the surgery. Many insurance plans require it, and you will feel better knowing that you looked at your problem from more than one perspective.

7. Find out about your insurance coverage and medical leave provisions. Nasty surprises in the form of unexpected medical bills or losing your job are not what women need when recovering from hysterectomy.

8. Assess your family situation. Can your husband and children get along without you while you are recuperating? Can they take care of themselves in the unlikely event something should happen to you?

9. Call on your supportive network. My family, my boyfriend, friends and coworkers were a blessing. I knew I would not be going through this experience alone.

10. Answer *for yourself* the fundamental questions: "How miserable is my current situation making me?" and "Do I want to continue living in this way?" Ultimately, I made my decision to have a hysterectomy without feeling pressured by any

outside source. Using all the information and evidence available to me, including the effect my condition was having on my lifestyle, I determined that I was miserable enough to take the radical step of having my uterus removed.

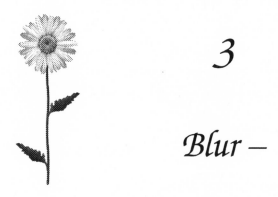

3

Blur –

Getting Ready For Surgery

~ ~ ~ ~ ~ ~ ~ ~ ~ ~ ~ ~ ~ ~ ~ ~ ~ ~ ~ ~

Rush hour was winding down, although the freeway was still crowded. Light rain dripped on the windshield as I sped along at sixty plus miles per hour. The drizzle outside was minor compared to the storm taking place inside me.

"Oh, God," I moaned.

"No, this can't happen!"

"I'm so scared," I shouted, shaking the steering wheel and trying to concentrate on the road through the blur of tears.

I was terrified that I would not wake up.

Tension had been building since my decision to have a hysterectomy, until it finally overwhelmed me, at a most inopportune place and time. The upcoming operation surged from being a backdrop against which all other activ-

~ ~

ities took place, to the top of my consciousness, where it had completely commandeered my emotions. I was convinced the lights would go out and never come back on again.

My rational voice reminded me I was in far more danger driving down a rainy road blinded by tears and terror than I faced during surgery. I managed to calm down enough to get to my destination.

The episode on the freeway encapsulated my feelings during the three weeks between the decision to have a hysterectomy and the surgery itself. I alternated between my usual "rise-to-the occasion" approach to any situation and my growing fear of the unknown.

In other words, I was a mess.

So Much To Do

On the one hand, having finally made a decision, I was impatient to proceed with the surgery. Among other things, I was thinking ahead to my son's being best man for his friend. I also looked forward to summertime, Michigan's best season, and I wanted to be able to resume most of my activities by the time Memorial Day came around.

On the other hand, compressing what is, by its very nature, a high-anxiety situation into such a short period of time merely elevated the stress.

There was a blur of things that had to be accomplished — appointments with the urologist, the pre-surgical work-up at the hospital, another session with Dr. Finn, plus a myriad of personal matters to attend to.

~ ~

A real complicating factor was my employment. The project I had been involved in for months was finally coming to fruition in late March, in the time period between my decision and the date of the actual surgery. I had to be in Southern California for nearly a week to help facilitate a major conference; I knew from experience it would be a time of high demands and little sleep.

DONATING MY OWN BLOOD

I was able to take care of one important matter before leaving town. Dr. Finn had given me the necessary forms for making an autologous blood donation through the Red Cross. Typically, hysterectomy does not require a transfusion, but there is always a possibility of excessive bleeding or complications, and we agreed it was best to be prepared.

The idea behind autologous donation is simple and extremely sensible in this era of HIV and other blood-related infections: Have your own blood drawn in advance of surgery, to be given back to you if a transfusion is needed.

The Red Cross people were friendly and understanding. They also provided additional proof that I was making the right decision.

The hemoglobin test showed, once again, that my red blood count was lower than it should have been — no doubt a legacy of my four-week-long period, which at that time was still going on. The nurse said she would have refused me had I simply come in to donate. Since I was leaving blood for myself, she agreed to go ahead. Dr. Finn had already prescribed an iron supplement to prepare me for the surgery, so my body could build itself up in time.

One item completed. I crossed it off my very long list.

SOMETHING NICE FOR MYSELF

Sometime before my business trip to California, I realized that I was going to be more or less in the vicinity of southwestern Utah. My former boss had retired to that area, and I had been wanting for at least a year and a half to take advantage of the open invitation to visit him and his wife. Once the hysterectomy began to look like a certainty, I was determined to do something nice for myself beforehand, and this was it.

I called John and Martha. Yes, they were going to be home at that time; yes, they would love to see me. I made arrangements to leave the weekend before I was due in California and stop over in Utah.

The visit was all I had hoped it would be. We marveled at the drama of Zion National Park, we speculated about the lives of our forbearers as we examined Native American petroglyphs, we shared good food and warm friendship as we toured and talked and enjoyed.

I learned that Martha had undergone a hysterectomy ten years before, when she was about my age. She was extremely open and generous about sharing her experience with me, and we talked at length. That helped, as I continued to struggle with doubt about the wisdom of my decision and fear about the upcoming surgery. Her circumstances had been somewhat different from mine, in that her surgery had been a medical emergency in the making, a do-it-now or you'll-end-up-doing-it-later-under-more-urgent-circumstances kind of deal. She had not been able to take synthetic hormones, so despite going into instant menopause with the removal of her ovaries and experiencing a year or so of discomfort as her body made the adjustment, she confirmed that having the surgery had been a wise choice. I felt a little better.

Most important, I relaxed, which was something I desperately needed to do. I also felt I had indulged myself just a bit.

A good thing, since the business portion of my trip was extremely hectic and pressured. I tried not to let what was facing me affect my work, but thoughts of the upcoming surgery were always there, lurking around the edges of my primary activity, manifesting themselves despite my best efforts. Occasional snappiness with colleagues and impatience when work did not progress as quickly as I thought it should were symptoms of my unease. Fortunately, the conference was a huge success. I flew home, exhausted after having gotten about nine hours of sleep over the course of three nights, and exhilarated at a job well done.

BACK TO THE BLADDER, ETC.

Dr. Clarence Andrews was a real surprise. Tall and trim, in his mid-thirties, with thick, dark, curly hair, I would have placed him in a more glamorous medical specialty than urology. He was personable and thoroughly professional.

He started my appointment by getting a personal history, during which I described, with some embarrassment, how frequently I wet myself. It had gotten to the point that when running or doing aerobics, I always had to wear a bladder protection pad, even though I went to the bathroom

immediately before starting the activity. If I laughed
heartily, I always had to pay attention to trying to hold onto
my urine, even if I was sitting down. When I had to sneeze,
I tightened my vaginal and thigh muscles to keep from
leaking. If I needed to sneeze while walking, I had to stop
and cross my legs before it happened, or walk around damp
for the next hour or so. And there were times when I had to
urinate so badly I simply could not control myself and
began to release the flow before I could get to the bathroom.

A pelvic exam was next, to test my bladder-retention
ability. At the doctor's cue, I coughed. And I leaked. After
more questions and examination, he determined that my
leakage was indeed due to stress incontinence (there are a
number of other conditions and infections that can cause
urinary problems). While my case was not extreme, it was,
in his judgment, sufficient to warrant adding a bladder
suspension to my surgical list. Fortunately, he had already
received the tentative surgery date from Dr. Finn and had
managed to rearrange his schedule to accommodate me.

Next, Dr. Andrews described the particular surgical
procedure he expected to use (there are different types of
suspensions possible) and laid out his post-surgery recovery
regime. He was considerably more restrictive than Dr. Finn:
No driving for four weeks, no impact exercise for three
months, no sex for eight weeks. "What about my poor
boyfriend?" I wailed at that final restriction. "If he's any
good, he'll wait," was the reply.

Actually I was more concerned about the forced
celibacy than Kal was. I knew intellectually that he was not
going to be troubled by the hiatus; emotionally was another
matter. At that level I tapped into primitive suspicions that
good sex was a way a woman "holds" her man. Without sex,

~ ~

I wondered, would he leave? Would he find somebody else? As an educated woman, I knew that was absurd. Yet, I worried, as many women facing hysterectomy do. The fact that I did not know how I would feel about sex when I was allowed to be active again was especially scary. Would taking away my uterus, and possibly my ovaries, take away my desire?

ABOUT URINARY STRESS INCONTINENCE AND BLADDER SUSPENSION

Stress incontinence is caused by the partial incompetence of the urinary sphincter, the muscle that controls the release of urine from the bladder. The condition most commonly manifests itself in the involuntary loss of urine when coughing, straining, sneezing, lifting or conducting any maneuver that suddenly increases intra-abdominal pressure. In women, stress incontinence is most commonly due to shortening of the urethra, the tube that carries urine from the bladder outside the body and loss of the normal angle of the organ resulting from pelvic relaxation. The most common causes of pelvic relaxation are aging and multiple childbirths; running and other impact exercise can also contribute to the condition.

A diagnosis of stress incontinence is established by a physician, using history, pelvic examination and demonstration of loss of urine by coughing or straining, which may be stopped by manipulation of the vaginal tissue.

Mild cases may respond to a series of muscle exercises. More severe cases require surgical correc-

> *tion, using one of several techniques. Basically, the surgery involves strengthening support for the bladder by reattaching or suspending it from ligaments inside the lower abdomen.*

OOPHORECTOMY ANYONE?

Having finally decided to have a hysterectomy, now I found myself battered by another stormy debate — should I have my ovaries out or would I be better off leaving them in my body, right where they had always been?

Looking for guidance, I once again started reading and talking to other women. And if I thought there was disagreement over the ifs and whys of hysterectomy, the ovary question was even worse.

The best estimate is that 40 to 50 percent of hysterectomies include removal of the tubes and ovaries (bilateral salpingo oophorectomy in medical parlance, if both sets of ovaries and tubes are taken out). In most cases, the ovaries removed are healthy. For women under the age of 45 who undergo hysterectomy, the rate of oophorectomy is lower.

So what's the big deal?

The answer to that question lies in the complex way female anatomy works.

I already knew, of course, that the ovaries produce the hormones responsible for governing the female cycle throughout the reproductive years: Estrogen to tell the endometrium, the lining of the uterus, when it was time to build itself up in preparation for a possible pregnancy; progesterone, when the egg released by the ovaries was not fertilized, causing a monthly period as the endometrium was ordered to break up and discharge.

I also knew that my hormones were important for reasons far beyond regulating the monthly cycle. Estrogen, in particular, plays a major role in protecting women against heart disease and osteoporosis, as well as influencing everything from the glow of our skin to the fluctuations of our sexual desire. In addition to female hormones, our ovaries produce small amounts of testosterone and several other male hormones, which enhance our libidos and may also contribute to an overall sense of well-being.

But as we age, the production of hormones tapers off and eventually ceases. We enter menopause, when our periods go away — which, for most of us, is the good news. The bad news is our risk of heart disease and damaging osteoporosis, which makes our bones brittle, increases dramatically, and we experience a range of other symptoms related to loss of estrogen. These symptoms manifest as everything from vaginal dryness to saggy breasts to loss of elasticity in our skin. In other words, without estrogen, we start to look and feel old.

Until fairly recently, perhaps 30 years ago, removal of the ovaries as part of hysterectomy was pretty much standard operating procedure. Women who were not menopausal at the time of surgery got that way — instantly. The sudden loss of their ovaries induced such immediate reactions as severe depression and complete loss of sexual desire. All too often, when these unfortunate women complained to their doctors (who, at that time, were almost exclusively male), the latter merely shrugged and advised their patients that whatever they were feeling was all in their own heads.

Fortunately, those days are, by and large, behind us. In the past few decades, medical science has taught us and our doctors a lot about the ovaries, including the fact that surgical removal of the organs while a women is still using them has severe consequences.

How severe depends on who is doing the talking.

The American College of Obstetricians and Gynecologists, in *Understanding Hysterectomy,* treats the question matter-of-factly.

"If the ovaries also are removed with the uterus prior to menopause, there are hormone-related effects. These effects may usually be treated satisfactorily through estrogen therapy."

At the other extreme is Nora Coffey of the HERS Foundation. She describes oophorectomy as female castration. *(HERS Newsletter,* vol. 2 no. 4)

"If the ovaries are removed in a premenopausal woman, an abrupt process termed 'surgical menopause' occurs. The process is more severe than normal menopause as the body has no time to gradually adjust to the loss of these hormones. Loss of libido (sexual desire), hot flashes, depressing weight gain, headaches, fatigue, vaginal dryness and thinning, and backaches are some of the symptoms that result from physical hormone disruptions."

I certainly did not want any of that. Still, I knew that many doctors routinely recommend removal of the ovaries for any woman over the age of 45. The reason is almost always to eliminate the possibility of ovarian cancer, which we can develop even after we enter menopause and our

~ ~

ovaries are largely inactive. The risk, in fact, increases as we age.

At the same time, other medical professionals argue that no woman should have her healthy ovaries taken out, regardless of her age. A third group advocates basing the decision on a woman's individual menopausal status and family history, since ovarian cancer exhibits a strong genetic link.

For younger women, the choice is generally quite clear: if the ovaries are healthy and functioning normally, leave them alone. (A possible exception is when hysterectomy is done for severe endometriosis, which is aggravated by estrogen.)

But at the age of 50, and surely approaching natural menopause, I could hardly count myself a "younger woman." So, I debated — and vacillated — what was the right thing for me to do?

WHAT ABOUT MY OVARIES?

I went back and forth many times.

The arguments for having my ovaries removed were persuasive: Obviously, I was nearing menopause, when my ovaries would become inactive. In addition, I had exhibited a growth on one of my ovaries, which may or may not have been more than a simple cyst.

Ovarian growths or tumors, can be, and most often are, benign and periodic, appearing and going away in relationship to a woman's menstrual cycle. For a persistent benign growth, either the affected tissue or the ovary is removed. If the growth is malignant, everything goes; ovaries, tubes and uterus, because of the possible micro-

~ ~

scopic, local spread of cancer. If a tumor shows some malignant characteristics but is not clearly a cancer, many physicians prefer to be safe and remove both ovaries, especially
in women who no longer wish to have children. For younger
women, who want to preserve fertility, it may be possible to
remove only the affected ovary and monitor the situation
closely for further signs of trouble.

Unfortunately, there is no way to determine whether
an ovarian growth is benign or malignant without examination of a tissue sample. That meant, at the very least in my
case, that if my cyst persisted, I would need a biopsy.

Talk of a biopsy led me to a consideration of ovarian
cancer. Though not a common disease (20,000 new cases
are reported annually in the U.S., or about 1 percent of the
female population), it is devastating when it does strike,
producing a fatality rate of at least 66 percent. Ovarian
cancer is particularly deadly because, unlike breast and
cervical malignancies, there is no means of early detection.
However, compared to breast cancer, which strikes one
woman in ten, ovarian cancer is quite rare.

The arguments for keeping my ovaries were just as
persuasive. Most obvious was the fact I was still using them.
I was not in menopause yet, and I did not know how soon I
would get there. Even after menopause, the ovaries continue
to produce small amounts of hormones, especially andro-
gens, and I certainly was not willing to eliminate sexual
desire and activity from my life. I also knew the increased
risks to post-menopausal women from heart disease, osteoporosis and other maladies related to loss of estrogen and I
was in no hurry to increase my chances in that regard.

Then there was the matter of aging. I did not feel old,
I did not want to look old quite yet, and I feared that losing

~ ~

my ovaries could hasten that particular transformation. I knew that having my ovaries removed would initiate instant menopause, which would affect my entire persona — moods, emotions, productivity, appearance, vitality. If I had the oophorectomy, what would happen to all of these traits? And what about hormone replacement therapy? I knew I would start on synthetic hormones immediately, but I had heard plenty of horror stories about women who could not tolerate hormones and women who gained weight and women who still lost their interest in sex. I also knew that many questions persist about the effects of long-term hormone replacement therapy, especially in relationship to breast and other cancers, and that research results were contradictory.

I asked other women what they had done. Some, including my mother, had kept their ovaries. That was especially true of women who were younger than I at the time of surgery. Others, such as my friend Martha, had had their ovaries removed. Most of the removal group had adjusted to synthetic hormones easily, but there was always the chance that I, like Martha, would not.

I talked to my sister. She is nearly eleven years younger than I am, so her perspective on the matter was different from mine. "At my age," she said, "I'd have to think a long time about having the ovaries removed unless there was some clear medical reason for it. I'm going to need them for a decade or so yet. But," she added, "at your age, I wouldn't hesitate, mostly because of ovarian cancer. I've seen it and it's incredibly awful; at least you can remove that risk."

I asked Dr. Finn, point blank, what she would do if faced with this decision. Although my junior by five years, she did not hesitate. "I'd have them out," she said.

She was also straightforward about the limitations of synthetic hormones. "The ovaries are highly complex organs with many functions. Even the best replacement hormones aren't as good as your own," she indicated. "We adjust the dosage to your needs, but it's a set amount, which means it can't fluctuate to respond to what's happening in your body like your natural hormones would." Not exactly a ringing endorsement.

I flip-flopped on the oophorectomy right up until the day of the surgery. I finally decided to go with the more conservative side of the medical establishment and forestall the possibility of ovarian cancer, even though I had no family history of the disease. I also knew, because of my constant PMS and sore breasts and general moodiness, that my own hormones had become erratic in their production and could be partially responsible for the constant bleeding and emotional turmoil that plagued me. At least synthetic hormones would smooth that out.

As it turned out, the decision was probably the correct one, although I have to admit that this is the one aspect of my surgery where I have had second thoughts. When Dr. Finn got inside me, she found a growth, a hemorrhagic cyst on my left ovary; my left fallopian tube was blocked with fluid, and there was scarring consistent with endometriosis. Apparently things were more of a mess in there than either of us had thought.

~ ~

OTHER WOMEN'S OVARIES

In talking with other women about this book, I found about half had kept their ovaries and half had had them removed.

Those who decided to forego oophorectomy tended, as is typical, to be younger than those who lost them. By keeping their ovaries, these women knew they were avoiding instant menopause; they also felt that because their ovaries were not causing them problems, they were wise to leave them in place. Although aware of ovarian cancer, these women did not feel themselves to be significantly at risk.

The women who did part with their ovaries generally were older and closer to natural menopause, or exhibited either abnormalities or a family history of ovarian problems. The medical professionals, in particular, were extremely wary of ovarian cancer, despite the small statistical possibility they might be at risk.

"Ovarian cancer is one of the scariest diagnoses you can come up with," said Helen, head nurse on a woman's care unit that deals with such conditions on a regular basis. "I've seen it, and I didn't have to think about having my ovaries out. My family has a history of cancer, although not this kind; it's terrible to even think about the possibility. My hormones weren't normal anymore anyway. I had terrible PMS, to the point that my family just tiptoed around me most of the time. And the hot flashes were so bad I actually had to get up and change my gown during the night."

Helen was 47, with two children when she had her surgery, which included a bladder suspension to correct the

~ ~

same kinds of problems with coughing or laughing that I had.

One of the younger women I spoke with, who did have her ovaries removed at age 37, also described having bad PMS. "My hormones were all messed up for the last year before I had the surgery. I don't know how my kids and my husband lived in the same house with me. I could describe myself in a very ugly way." This from Lea, an outgoing, ebullient woman who also listed a family history of various female problems — both her mother and sister had had hysterectomies. "I had a small spot of something on one of my ovaries," she added, "so even though I was fairly young to have them out, I never gave it a second thought."

Another woman, Victoria, 50 years old, had yet a different experience. "My gynecologist didn't really tell me there was no good way to detect ovarian cancer until it's too late; my regular doctor did. So I went back to my gynecologist and said I'd just as soon have my ovaries out, too. I knew I wouldn't miss my up-and-down hormone production and the mood swings. I was so tense, I went around with my jaw clenched a lot of the time."

As with so many other aspects of hysterectomy, removal of the ovaries ultimately comes down to a very personal and often, very ambiguous decision. While a woman is well advised to seek the counsel of her physician, finally, she has to decide what's right for her. Family history, and certainly medical indications of abnormality, must be carefully evaluated. And even for a woman who seems to be at no special risk of ovarian cancer, sheer peace of mind can be sufficient reason to have the ovaries removed. It's a very individual choice.

~ ~

MORE PRE-SURGERY REQUIREMENTS

Everybody needed to see me.

The hospital wanted me in for a pre-surgery workup. Blood tests, electrocardiogram, discussion of anesthesia, religious preferences — they asked all the questions and poked me full of holes. I read and signed the Patient's Rights statement. I read and signed the surgical consent forms. Dr. Andrews wanted an ultrasound of my kidneys to check for any problems there. I got that done. Thankfully, the hospital personnel were friendly, efficient and understanding. Not having to wait in tedious lines was particularly helpful, especially since my stress level was continuing to rise, and patience, even under normal circumstances, had never been my most abundant quality.

Dr. Finn wanted to do a D and C prior to the hysterectomy. With my ongoing bleeding, she needed to forestall any nasty surprises once we got to surgery by checking on causes other than fibroids. But she found my uterus so distended and misshapen she could not insert the instruments. We settled for an endometrial biopsy, which was a less extensive measure, and just fine with me. More evidence that hysterectomy might be the right thing for me to do.

Dr. Andrews needed to perform cystoscopy to look inside my bladder for abnormalities. Another appointment, another procedure. When I arrived for that one, his office was jammed with patients — an earlier emergency left him running ninety minutes behind schedule. That delay gave me time to go to a nearby mall to do some shopping; Kal's birthday was a week after my surgery and I knew I was not going to be going shopping then.

As I entered the final days before surgery, I was trying to plan ahead, anticipate every detail, do the dozens of things that normally would be spread out over weeks. I made long lists of tasks to be accomplished. At times it seemed that I added new items more quickly than I could cross others off.

Among other things, realizing that I was about to undergo major surgery, "where there is a risk of something going wrong," as the medical profession so euphemistically puts it, I pulled out my will and looked at it. Woefully out of date. I called my attorney and scrambled around updating the document. I signed the revised papers about 18 hours before the surgery — but I got it done.

There were friends to call. Grandchildren to hug. Arrangements to be made. Did I have the right things packed to take to the hospital? Would I remember to take the autologous blood donation form with me and leave my jewelry at home? Did I have enough pads to handle the bleeding after surgery? Had I taken care of everything at the office? I paid my bills. I called American Express to tell them I would be out of circulation since they do not like to wait for their payments. I got as specific as stocking up on enough cat food to feed my felines for the several weeks I would not be able to get to the store.

Anticipating a quick descent after surgery into boredom, I bought or borrowed a dozen books. I got my hair cut. I kept my exercise schedule, even though I was pressed for time, because I knew working out kept my stress level down. In the final days, I savored a last swim, run, and session of aerobics, unsure how soon I would be able to enjoy those activities again. Kal and I made love one last time. As he lay sleeping beside me, I wondered if our pleasure in one another would ever be the same again.

There was one other issue to deal with — where to go when I got out of the hospital. My daughter and grandsons were living at my house at that time, waiting to get into their new residence. Having a four-year-old and a two-year-old around did not seem very conducive to my recuperation. The boys were not undisciplined or rowdy; they were just exuberant pre-schoolers, accustomed to being able to climb all over grandma at any time. Once again, Kal came to the rescue. He invited me to stay with him for a while, with nothing to do but read and sleep and watch television. That was a godsend, for me and for my daughter and the boys.

IMAGING THE POSITIVE

I got through the days because they were frenzied with activity. The rational side of my brain made the lists, organized tasks, tried to anticipate every need.

The nights were another matter. That was when the emotional side took over. I lay wide-eyed, sweaty with anxiety and hot flashes. The Oh-God-I-might-not-wake-up terror reasserted itself in the frightening hours before dawn. Often I would fall asleep exhausted from the day's schedule, only to awaken after a few hours, unable to get back to sleep. Some nights I tried reading until I dozed off; other nights I just flipped from side to back to side again, unable to relax enough to fall asleep.

After enduring several of my sleepless nights, Kal suggested an alternative — imaging. The idea was to replace negative, fear-inducing mental pictures with positive, happy ones. I was willing to try it. Since we were already planning an August vacation to the Pacific Northwest, I used my mind's eye to place us at Cape Flattery, at the northwest tip of Washington's Olympic Peninsula. Cape Flattery is the absolute end of the land, a high bluff overlooking the Pacific, surrounded by dramatic sea stacks and undercut by deep caves and charging surf. Beyond this wild precipice stretches nothing but ocean, for thousands of miles.

It worked. In the days before the surgery, I called up that image many times, not only lying in bed at night, but during the daytime when I felt myself growing especially tense and strung out.

I also visited with the pastor at church. My wanting to seek strength and comfort from a religious source "surprised the hell out of me," as I told him. I had been married to a clergyman and after the divorce, I stayed away from any sort of organized religion for twenty years. Only recently had I ventured near a church again, and then to one of a different denomination. As it turned out, the pastor's wife had had a hysterectomy some years earlier. He reassured me that everything had gone fine for her and that their relationship had actually gotten stronger as a result of her improved health.

OTHER WOMEN'S FEARS

In recalling how fearful I was before surgery, I wondered if I was unduly frightened, perhaps because I had never had surgery of this magnitude before. So I asked other women about their pre-surgery anxieties.

As with so many other aspects of hysterectomy, their reactions were mixed.

~ ~

Despite the fact that hysterectomy usually entails a general anesthetic, often requires an abdominal incision and at the very least involves removal of one major internal organ and rearrangement of what is left, some women rolled into surgery with hardly a second thought. In many cases, they felt they were able to do so because they had been well prepared by their doctors. "My doctor actually called me at home the night before my operation," reported one fortunate woman. "And she spent about forty-five minutes talking to me in great detail about everything I could expect to happen. That really helped me."

All women should be so lucky.

Others facing surgery, especially those with medical backgrounds, freely admitted being scared. "As a nurse, I think it was even worse for me," said one. "Because going into surgery, I *knew* everything that could go wrong."

She added, "Anytime you're working with general anesthetic, there is a risk."

Said another, "I'm in the medical profession, I'm a human being and I was scared."

Yet another reported: "I was afraid I was going to die; I was afraid I'd have an allergic reaction; I was afraid some doctor, especially the anesthesiologist, would screw up and I'd never wake up."

Which is not an unfounded fear, as it turns out, since many of the deaths that do occur during hysterectomies can be traced to anesthesia. Unexpected, uncontrollable bleeding is the other most common cause of death.

What all of this underscores is that hysterectomy, and accompanying procedures, should not be undertaken lightly. No surgery should be, especially one that entails entering the abdominal cavity and removing the organs that define our reproductive systems and our femininity. The physical trauma to the body is very real.

THE NIGHT BEFORE

The chores were completed, the lists of things to do were finished and every detail I could think of had been covered. Kal and I went to get something to eat — long before midnight, since that was my deadline for eating or drinking before surgery. I had been instructed to cut out alcohol as of two days before.

I was bleeding again, even though my last period, the four-week-long one, had ended only ten days before. And cramps! These were bad ones, so severe I could hardly stand up straight. My elevated pre-surgery stress probably increased the pain; maybe my ovaries were giving me one last shot of natural hormones, just so I had something to remember them by. When we got back to the house, I gave Kal an envelope that contained a copy of my revised will and some cash for my daughter. I wanted him to be prepared to handle the details should something awful happen. And I asked him to "sniff" my forehead — a love gesture we have shared since our first weeks together — the next morning before they wheeled me away.

With everything in order, snuggled next to the man I loved, I actually slept fairly well.

~ ~

WHAT WAS IMPORTANT

My recommendations regarding pre-surgery preparation.

1. Make sure everything is in order. In my case that included notifying family and friends, laying in a supply of books, updating my will, making sure everything was covered at the office and attending to a host of other details. To make sure I did not forget anything important, I made lists for myself and followed them until everything was done.

2. Do something nice for yourself before surgery, if possible, and anticipate what might make you feel better afterward, as well. I was fortunate to be able to schedule the trip to see old friends. Other women filled their homes with flowers and plants or planned trips to vacation cottages because they knew these were things that were important to them.

3. Keep as physically fit as possible. I maintained regular exercise, even though I was extremely pressed for time, because I knew it helped me keep my stress under control. I also found my physical strength was an asset during recuperation — strong arms and legs helped me accomplish such basics as getting in and out of bed.

4. Clear the decks for the weeks after surgery. I tried to anticipate every detail, from paying bills in advance to getting enough cat food to last four weeks to getting my hair cut and telling the cleaning service when not to come. I suspected I

~ ~

would need to concentrate all my energies in those first weeks on recovery, and I was right.

5. Find things to look forward to after recovery. Using imaging to make the mental leap to a time when I would be feeling good again helped me deal with my more immediate fears.

6. Find ways to stay calm. Exercise was important, as I have indicated. Talking to other women who had had hysterectomies, seeking counsel from my pastor, spending time with my children, grandchildren and friends were also sources of comfort.

Part II

How To Survive

There is a clear timeline associated with surgery and recovery, with definite milestones along the way. Here each phase is examined in detail.

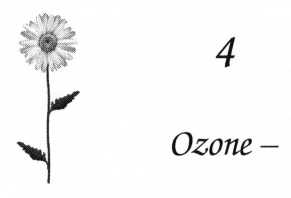

4

Ozone –

One To Two Weeks

~ ~ ~ ~ ~ ~ ~ ~ ~ ~ ~ ~ ~ ~ ~ ~ ~ ~ ~ ~

One halting step after another, I made my way to the bathroom. Towel, clean underwear, clean tee shirt — yes, I had everything I needed. Having to walk back to the bedroom to get anything I had forgotten would have been just too hard.

Slowly, gingerly, I removed my shirt, preparing to take my first shower since leaving the hospital. I leaned on the edge of the counter for support.

"Oh, my God!" I gasped as I saw my first full length reflection in the mirror.

I already knew that my face looked gaunt and drawn. But now I realized with near-horror that my ribs protruded from my midsection and my arms and legs looked like weak sticks. Worst was the pallor of my skin; from hairline to toenails, I had the grayish color of library paste.

With shock, I got a good look at my incision. The mirror showed a slash just above my pubic hair, six inches long, still in the process of scabbing over, with a single black stitch visible at the right end. A fold of skin draped limply over the incision, excess tissue now that my swollen uterus was gone.

For the first time, I realized how downright awful I looked. And I felt as rough as I appeared in the mirror.

At that moment the reality of my surgery finally hit home. Until then, I had not seen myself as others were seeing me. I had not been fully aware of the physical changes this insult to my body had produced.

AUTOMATIC PILOT MEETS BLACK HOLE

I was awake early the day of the surgery, before the alarm went off. Even though it was the sixth of April, I looked out the window to find several inches of sloppy spring snow. I was due at the hospital at 8:00 a.m. for 9:30 a.m. surgery. Kal had rearranged his schedule to spend the day with me, and we arrived a few minutes late, delayed by weather and traffic. It did not matter much; everybody else was late that day, too.

From that point on, things progressed rapidly. I felt a kind of numb detachment as I was prepped for surgery. Fortunately, the procedure was quick and efficient, the staff friendly, understanding, and thoroughly professional. That helped me feel as confident as possible under the circumstances. Within thirty minutes of my check-in, I was stretched out on a gurney, with an intravenous needle stuck

~ ~

in the back of my left hand. Shortly thereafter I began to get groggy, relaxed by some sort of drug intended to mellow out my very ragged edges. Since I could not eat or drink anything (I had brushed my teeth, careful not to swallow the water), I could not take anything for the raging cramps that were twisting my innards.

When it was time to go to surgery, Kal walked down the hall beside me, holding my hand. He sniffed me, as promised, we exchanged "I love you's," then he was gone.

I was pushed into a room with a dozen other patients. Lying stretched out, gurney to gurney, all gowned and IV'ed, we waited. My surgery was supposed to start at 9:30, but at 10:00 I was still in the holding area. Apparently the doctor doing a prior surgery in the operating room for which I was scheduled had been delayed by the weather. Although I was groggy, I was at the stage where I just wanted to get it over with. Finally, at about 10:15 a.m., the attendant moved me out of the holding room, across the hall and into the bright lights of Operating Theatre #3.

Quickly, I was lifted from the gurney onto the table, my arms outstretched to either side and secured. A surprising number of people were already in the room, busily attending to tasks that I could only assume had something to do with me.

The anesthetist began his work by asking me if I wanted to see Dr. Finn before he put me under. I managed a weak affirmative. I was determined to make sure I was in the right place with the right doctor before anybody started cutting. I imagined I could still leap off the table and bring things to halt if the wrong surgeon showed up.

Dr. Finn appeared — masked, gloved, in green scrubs — and greeted me. For some strange reason, the last thing I

~ ~

remember thinking was: Gee, she's a lot shorter than I thought. Then — black hole!

General anesthesia was a weird and scary sensation. This was only the third time in my life I had had a general, and each time made me increasingly uneasy. Unlike sleeping, anesthesia blocks out all awareness of surrounding sounds and activities, which, of course, was what it is supposed to do. It was the complete and utter gap in memory, the total disconnection from reality and personality, that I found disquieting. Dr. Finn said that the longer patients are out, the greater the risk of psychotic-like complications later. I could begin to understand that, because surely death must be something like general anesthesia. Except that this time I got to wake up.

For several weeks after the operation, I relived as a nightmare those last few moments before going under. Even months later, I felt dread, fear, even the urge to cry when I thought about the actual surgery, for reasons that I do not consciously understand. I do have a vague, unfocused recollection of speaking to someone while I was out, or more likely as I was awakening in recovery. I read later that patients sometimes partially awake during surgery and complain of pain, but when I asked her, Dr. Finn said she was not aware of any problems along that line. Perhaps I did experience a greater level of awareness during surgery than I was intended to. I'll never know for sure.

The first clear memory I have following surgery was being wheeled into my hospital room and transferred from the gurney to a bed. Kal was there, smiling "Hi, Honey" to me, and holding my hand.

I was awake! I was alive! I hurt like hell! Thank God.

~ ~

ABOUT SURGICAL PROCEDURE IN ABDOMINAL HYSTERECTOMY

Before actual surgery begins, administration of anesthesia is accomplished, using a tube inserted through the mouth into the trachea and lungs for general anesthetic. The vaginal area is cleaned and a sterile Foley catheter placed in the urethra. Following cleansing and draping of the abdomen, a Pfannenstiel or bikini line incision is made in the lower abdomen and carried through the skin layers. Blood vessels are clamped and cauterized after being cut. Muscles are dissected. Once the peritoneum, the protective lining of the abdomen, is reached, it is opened with a scalpel and extended as needed to accommodate the size of the uterus to be removed.

In removing the uterus, and the ovaries, if the latter are included in the procedure, the ligaments holding the organ are severed and sutured (stitched). Blood vessels are severed and sutured. Finally, the uterus itself is cut free. The cervix is then freed from attachment to the vagina and the top of the vagina sutured to create a rounded closure where the cervix had been. The ovaries are cut free from ligaments and blood vessels and removed in a similar manner. Following cleansing of the abdominal cavity, and removal and counting of needles, sponges and other instruments, the peritoneum, muscles and layers of skin are sutured closed.

ABOUT SURGICAL ALTERNATIVES

As with so many other aspects of hysterectomy, a number of surgical variations are possible.

In some cases, if the uterus is small, the organ may be removed without an abdominal cut, through the vagina. Although becoming more common, especially since the introduction in 1991 of laparascopically-assisted procedures, vaginal hysterectomies still account for only about a quarter of the total performed.

Generally, surgery is performed while the patient is under general anesthesia. There are instances, however, when surgery is performed while the woman is awake, using a spinal or epidural anesthetic to block feeling below a certain point in the body. Two such stories are told here. Both patients were medical professionals; one a nurse and the other a physician.

Jody, the nurse, had a vaginal hysterectomy after three years of hemorrhaging and passing tennis ball-sized clots. Thirty-seven at the time of surgery, her healthy ovaries were left in place.

"My doctor chose to use a spinal anes-thetic, rather than a general. I sweat bullets about that for two weeks. When I first got in the operating room, the doctors were chatting and joking about stuff that had nothing to do with why we were all there. I was put off by that, especially since I was sitting on the edge of the table getting woozy because of the sedative in my IV. I felt like I was just surgery #178 in some huge assembly line, and I didn't like that. Later, though, during the actual procedure, the doctors talked to me and that helped calm me down. Once they got my uterus out, I wanted to see it.

So they showed me. All in all, it was a pretty positive experience. And I do know that by not having a general, I came back faster; general anesthetic affects your whole system and really slows you up."

Lynn had an even more amazing story: She was fairly young for a hysterectomy, 36, but she had very large fibroids and very heavy and increasingly suspicious bleeding.

"I'm a physician, so I want to have my hands in everything, especially when it relates to me. I insisted on being awake, and my gynecologist, who is fantastic, was willing to work with me. Part of the reason was we had to make decisions during the actual surgery as to what we were going to do. We used an epidural anesthesia, which works on the spinal cord to numb everything from that level down. I had an abdominal incision, which is unusual with a spinal. But the incision was necessary because of the massive size of what I had inside.

"At first we were going to try to just take out the fibroids, but that didn't work — they were just too extensive and were really pressing on my bladder. I also had a large, blood-filled cyst on my left ovary, and endometriosis everywhere. So we ended up taking everything out.

"It turned out to be a difficult procedure, and I lost a fair amount of blood — three units, to be exact. But I know my body well enough that I could actually be of assistance to the surgeon and the anesthesiologist.

"For example, I knew the body reacts to pain by a sharp drop-off in blood pressure.

~ ~

That's caused by the vagal nerve responding to the pain stimulus, and is usually followed by nausea. The last thing you want during surgery is the patient throwing up.

"At one point, the gynecologist tugged on my diaphragm, and despite the anesthetic, it hurt. I felt my heart rate drop, and told the anesthesiologist to watch out because my blood pressure was about to bottom out. He had time to ask me what in the world I was talking about, but he got ready. Bam! my pressure took the dive, fifteen or twenty seconds max after I felt the pain. The anesthesiologist was prepared with medication, my pressure stabilized and after that I went right on talking.

"After the surgery, we left the epidural in place until the next day to control the pain. I was wide awake in recovery because there had been no narcotic and no general sedation, so I wasn't groggy."

Asked about her rather singular experience, Lynn laughed as she reflected:

"No, I certainly don't recommend for most women to be awake. I know I drove them nuts being so talkative. Doing it that way requires a high level of patient cooperation, and a very strong stomach. I have to admit that, even with the epidural numbing me up, I got real uncomfortable several times. There was a lot of pulling and tugging and manipulation going on inside me. I'd grit my teeth, because I knew what was happening, but a couple of times it still took my breath away. That's why most doctors and hospitals prefer a general anesthetic — they

~ ~ ~ ~ ~ ~ ~ ~ ~ ~ ~ ~ ~ ~ ~ ~ ~ ~ ~ ~

don't believe the patient can be helpful to the procedure, and in most cases they may be right.

"The other real advantage for me was that I was up and around the next day and out of the hospital in 48 hours."

The brevity of Lynn's hospital stay was as atypical as her being an active participant in her surgery. Three to four days is more common for most women, down considerably from the full week that was common fifteen or twenty years ago.

HOSPITAL DAZE

During the three days and few odd hours I spent in the hospital, I learned several important lessons. The most important was: let them do everything; that's their job. My job was to do what I was told in the interest of getting better.

Actually, my memory of that time is very fuzzy. Wednesday evening, the day of the surgery, several friends stopped by to encourage me. Later, they referred to conversations in which they said I participated; I do not recall doing so, which was not surprising. I was substantially doped up.

I first learned about Patient Controlled Analgesia when my son had surgery for a serious back injury in 1988. The pump allows a patient to self-administer pain medication; maximum dosages are controlled, as is frequency. According to research, the pump has proved to be remarkably effective, with patients actually demanding less medication than when pain killers are given orally or by injection. Putting control in the patient's hands seemed to be the crucial factor.

After surgery, I was attached to such a pump, plus an IV, plus a catheter. Tubes were going in all directions — not a pretty sight.

The pump quickly became both a comfort and a frustration. On those occasions when I was allowed a dose, a reassuring "bleep" followed a press of the controller. Other times, when my pain level convinced me I was due more medication, I desperately thumbed the button. Nothing, not until the pump was good and ready, and the programming said "okay."

Attempting to make myself more comfortable, I did figure out several useful tricks. The most important was to take pressure off the incision, which meant not lying fully extended or flat on my back. Raising my knees (the electrically-controlled hospital bed made that easy) lessened the downward pull on the incision, easing the pain. I also found I was more comfortable lying slightly on one side with pillows behind me to support my back. That also shifted gravity away from my midsection. At first I had to ask for help in placing the pillows or turning from side to side; by the time I left the hospital I was able to accomplish those things myself. Once I was home, I continued to prop up my knees with cushions and lie on my side with my back supported for at least two more weeks. I simply felt better that way.

What didn't feel good at all was standing for the first time. Two nurses, one a solidly-built young man, arrived at my bedside the evening of the surgery and calmly informed me I was about to get to my feet. I told them they were crazy, and in a less-than-polite manner. They insisted, and moved to make me comply. One on either side, with gentle insistence, they swung my feet to the floor and got the rest of my body in position. A lift from both sides and I was actually standing. Pain, nausea and weakness immediately overwhelmed me. I nearly passed out. But the attendants were satisfied; I had actually stood, which was all I was supposed to do. They quickly got me back in bed, where I stayed until the next morning.

The cuisine of choice that first evening was ice chips. I tried apple juice, but it made me nauseated, and I went back to the ice. By the next morning I graduated to a semi-liquid diet — broth, jello, coffee — and from there, on the third day, to solid food. The hospital tried hard, but the food was typical institutional fare — bland, luke-cold and taste-less. At that point, gourmet meals were far down my list of immediate concerns. I was more interested in getting some sleep.

Sleep turned out to be another of those elusive hospital qualities. My first night was spent with a seriously ill roommate who required frequent attention. I was awakened from my own fitful slumber by nurses coming and going at least once every hour. The next morning I asked for, and got, a transfer to another room. Although the new roommate situation was more compatible, light and activity occurred at all hours of the night. Ironic that a place of supposed rest and recuperation offers patients very little of either.

Continuing my efforts at walking, I negotiated the room switch under my own power about 24 hours after surgery. Very slowly, leaning heavily on my son's arm, I walked down the hall and around the corner, using my own two feet. A small triumph, but I was proud of my accom-

~ ~

plishment. Actually, I was encouraged to walk and told to do it several times a day. The assignment seemed downright cruel.

The first challenge was actually getting out of bed. This proved to be a multi-phase process. The initial step was to roll onto my side and swing my feet over the edge of the bed. Then, I had to raise up my torso. In the hospital, I let the electric bed do that for me. Later, at home, I had to use my arms to push myself upright. (I had always hated doing pushups in aerobics class, but they paid off in upper body strength, which was suddenly very handy.) Strong leg muscles were the key to finally standing. From a sitting position on the edge of the bed, with feet slightly apart for balance, I used a determined push, relying on the legs and not my midsection, to get up.

Walking hurt and was awkward, especially while I was tethered to my IV pole. But I needed to get my blood flowing and persuade my muscles to work, so I kept trying. Walking did get easier each time. By Friday, when I was unhooked from the IV tubes and catheter lines, I walked around, very slowly, modeling my new, non-regulation hospital gown. The gown was an oversized nightshirt, imprinted front and back with a voluptuous female body dressed in a skimpy red teddy, with a garter belt and ribbons. I had spotted the shirt while doing some pre-surgery shopping, and figuring it might help to maintain a sense of humor, I bought it for hospital wear. Nurses and patients alike got a laugh out of the shirt; I even managed a smile.

Soon, plants, flowers and balloons began to brighten up my room. Kal presented me with the first bouquet right after surgery. It was the best possible way to wake up —

~ ~ ~ ~ ~ ~ ~ ~ ~ ~ ~ ~ ~ ~ ~ ~ ~ ~ ~ ~

seeing his smile above an armful of flowers. Then other contributions began arriving from family, friends and co-workers. These gifts were tangible evidence that people were thinking about me, and I was grateful. (The plants are at my home now, and I'm pleased to say, all of them continue to thrive.)

I learned very quickly that surgery is a great leveler. The most basic of bodily functions, including those we tend to ignore, take for granted or avoid discussing in polite company, suddenly command great attention and respect.

Like coughing. Unless I had a cold, I did not think much about coughing, but here I was instructed not just to think about it, but to do it, frequently. The very real purpose of coughing after surgery and general anesthesia was to clear the lungs and prevent pneumonia. There was only one problem — coughing hurt! As it turned out, coughing involves a lot of abdominal action, and my abdomen was in a very tender state. But I coughed, and was surprised to hear how much congestion had accumulated in my lungs.

And then there was sneezing. If coughing was painful, sneezing was downright agonizing, because it required a complicated series of abdominal activities. First, the inhale as the sneeze developed; then, the breath-holding pause as it gathered force; finally, the snapping jolt as the sneeze delivered — with different muscle and nerve combinations protesting mightily from beginning to end.

Fortunately, a nurse showed me a way to lessen the discomfort — simply hold the abdomen firmly and press slightly up and in. It worked; coughing and sneezing became at least bearable, although I tried everything possible to avoid sneezing for several weeks.

The same trick worked for laughing. Within two days of surgery, I found out why they call a rollicking guffaw a "belly laugh." Actually, all it took to engage the abdominal muscles was a mild titter, and even that hurt. For weeks whenever someone said something funny, I pleaded, "Don't make me laugh," and grabbed for my gut.

On a more basic level, a hospital is not the place to get easily embarrassed. Somebody is monitoring the most fundamental of bodily functions at all times. I was attached to a catheter for the first 48 hours, with periodic checks of my urinary output. When I was not producing enough, I was ordered to drink more fluids, which I did. After the catheter was removed, I had to report every time I went to the bathroom and precisely measure my production.

The return of normal urinary function was of particular concern because of my bladder suspension, and I still remember how slow and painful the first few voidings were. Making certain the bladder emptied fully after the suspension was important; undischarged urine can cause infection, at a time when an infection could develop into a major problem. Dr. Andrews had prepared me for the possibility of intermittent catheterization, which involved inserting a soft plastic tube into the urethra to finish emptying the bladder. He said I might have to keep doing that even after I went home. That sounded unpleasant to me, so I told my body before we went to the hospital that we were not going to have to do that; I was determined my bladder would function completely and normally on its own. The self-talk must have worked; the nurses performed the intermittent catheterization several times, and my bladder was so completely emptied they could not coax out a single extra drop.

~ ~

Detailed descriptions of my gastric and bowel activity were another requirement — did I feel any rumblings, was I passing gas, did I feel the urge to go to the bathroom? Hopefully, bowel function would resume on its own after a couple of days, I was told, and if it did not, nature would receive medicinal encouragement. Because of the incision, and all the recent internal activity in this region of my body, I was also warned not to push or strain. I felt utter triumph when the first movement actually happened, and over a function usually taken for granted. I was just so grateful that everything worked!

One of life's often overlooked small pleasures is the shower. I took my first one two days after the surgery, after all the tubes and lines and monitors had been removed. The shower chair was a welcome aid, since I was still wobbly and light-headed. The water was uncomfortable, beating on the incision; that particular sensation continued for the next three weeks. But clean hair and fresh skin did wonders for both body and spirit, and I began to feel like I might actually survive.

By and large the hospital staff was considerate and responsive, and my stay was about as decent as it could have been. Like so many facilities, this one was short of nursing personnel, and my asking for what I needed was the best way to get it. I tried to be as considerate as possible, although on one occasion I became demanding to get a problem solved. It was a simple matter: the line from the catheter to the bag got a kink that shut the tube, backing urine up in my bladder. I pushed the call button to summon a nurse. "Someone will be there shortly," an aide informed me over the intercom; "We're on a shift change and everyone is in conference." I waited several minutes,

~ ~

growing more uncomfortable. I called again and was
assured someone would very soon be on the way. More
minutes went by, with the discomfort turning into pain. I
tried calling one more time, with the same results. In
desperation I called the hospital operator and reported the
problem. That got action! Within ninety seconds two nurses
and an aide appeared at my bedside; none was pleased. I did
not like the possibility that I had caused someone trouble;
on the other hand, I did what I felt I needed to for my own
health.

I figured out several little ways to increase my sense
of comfort while at the hospital. Probably most important, I
had my daughter bring my pillow from home, which had
been molded to my personal contours through years of use.
I wore sweat socks the entire time I was in bed because the
combination of inactivity and trauma made my feet cold.
Long-sleeved tee shirts were great for protecting my
elbows; the roughness of hospital sheets laundered in harsh
disinfectants had rubbed my arms raw. Getting out of faded
hospital gowns and into my own night shirts was also an ego
booster; I felt a little more human wearing decent, familiar
things.

One of the nurses provided welcome reassurance
regarding my future appearance. Checking the newly-
acquired seam in my abdomen she pronounced it "a pretty
incision." "I've seen a lot of them," she added, "and this is
one of the best." Indeed it was, as these things go. The
closure was done like a French seam, with no visible
stitches, except one at the far right end of the cut. Within
three weeks that one had disappeared, dissolved along with
the seven layers of sutures that I could not see deep inside.

~ ~

Just three days and a few odd hours after my surgery, I went home. I left the hospital with flowers, plants, balloons and three prescriptions; one for pain, an antibiotic to prevent infection and my synthetic hormones. My discharge instructions included lots of rest, regular diet, no strenuous activity for six weeks, no creams or ointments on the incision, nothing in the vagina for eight weeks and no driving for two to three weeks. Despite the fact the oral pain medication was making me nauseated and lightheaded, and Dr. Finn's preference that I remain another day at the hospital, the insurance company had deemed it was time for me to go. As one of the nurses observed when I described how shaky and uncertain I still felt, "They know you feel miserable, but they figure you can be miserable at home."

Leaving the hospital, I found sunny, early spring weather with no trace of the snow that had fallen the day of the operation. After being cooped up in medicinal air next to other sick people, I was glad to be outside. With Kal on one side and an aide on the other, I managed to lower myself into the car seat; then they helped me swing my legs around. I leaned the seat back to take the pressure off my incision as we began the trip home. Kal drove carefully, but Michigan bumps and potholes were everywhere, and they seemed to reach up to jostle my aching body every chance they got.

EVERYTHING HURTS

From waist to pubic bone, hip to hip, I was sore! Every facet of my awareness was focused on my midsection; the most routine actions, like turning over in bed or reaching for the telephone, were a chore. Between the

~ ~

trauma of the surgery, the medications for pain and infection, the pain I was experiencing and the fact that this was
such a complete break from my normal routine, I felt
disconnected from myself and the world around me.

My job at this point was to avoid anything that looked,
felt or seemed like heavy activity. Kal's condo was the ideal
place to do that — no stairs, a compact layout with nothing
to detract me from getting lots of rest. The scene at my
house would have been much different: two boisterous
grandsons and my daughter in residence, kitchen on the first
floor, my bedroom on the second and reminders everywhere
of all the projects I needed to do.

Being a good Virgo (according to the astrologers, we
need structure), I quickly attached a routine to my days. Kal
left for work early, around 6:30 in the morning, after which
I went back to sleep. I would awaken again around 9:00
a.m., eat a light breakfast and read until my first daily high-
light at 11:00 a.m. — *Magnum, P.I.* reruns. Even in my
post-surgery haze, I lusted after Tom Selleck. That was
encouraging – at least I could still recognize a hunk when I
saw one, and he was a sensitive guy, too.

Not a great TV watcher when I was in good health, I
discovered daytime television was a whole other world. I
knew about the talk shows, of course, and the soap operas,
but having worked my entire adult life, I had never actually
watched any of these shows. I did not now either, even
though I knew many women in my condition would have
enjoyed them. For me, the convoluted plots of the soaps, the
outrageousness of the tabloid topics and the forced hyper-
activity of the talk shows were just too much.

And then there were the commercials! No car companies, no financial services, no McDonald's or Nike or Sears.

~ ~ ~ ~ ~ ~ ~ ~ ~ ~ ~ ~ ~ ~ ~ ~ ~ ~ ~ ~

Instead of the familiar prime time advertisers, I saw poorly-produced spots for several brands of psychics and a raft of personal injury lawyers, all promising big results for nominal fees. Quickie make-over/photo studios were popular, as were pitches for debt consolidation loans and get-a-great-job appeals from technical training schools. The whole tone of these commercials was different from what I was used to — they seemed to play off problems and hawked easy solutions to tough needs.

So I concentrated my TV viewing on reruns of favorite dramas and sitcoms. I also read a lot, although I discovered I could not handle anything dense or demanding. Mindless adventure, romantic page turners and travel books were my preference.

I would have lunch, take an afternoon nap and then wait to hear Kal's key in the lock, which was the real high-point of the day.

Having the man I loved take care of me was especially helpful to my recovery. Our roles underwent a classic reversal, with him doing the cooking, shopping, cleaning and generally fussing over me. Despite the extra work, he enjoyed having me to come home to; whenever I talked about returning to my house, he informed me I needed to stay around a while longer and keep resting. I was happy to do so, because for those first days, all my energy was concentrated on performing the most basic of functions. Besides Kal, my only contact with the outside world was the telephone, and talking, I quickly learned, was a major effort. For perhaps the first time in my adult life I was virtually isolated. For those initial days, that was just fine.

My first real effort at re-entering the land of the almost-human was seven days after the operation. It was

~ ~

Kal's birthday, and I wanted to create some semblance of a celebration for him. I had shopped for a gift during the period of pre-surgical frenzy and put the present at home where my daughter could easily find it. When she brought it over, I asked her to go to the grocery store and bring in dinner and a birthday cake. My grandsons bounded into Kal's with their usual energy; although I had to explain in preschool terms why grandma could not pick them up, their obvious glee at seeing me was a real lift.

By the time Kal came home, I had survived the shock of my first at-home shower, put on a new nightshirt, which was as flattering as possible under the circumstances, and applied make-up and lipstick for the first time in a week. The observance was certainly modest, but it felt like a step in the right direction. From that day on, I changed clothes and brightened myself up with lipstick every evening before Kal got home.

Sleeping and eating remained major preoccupations, and determining the best way to achieve them took some experimentation. I slept alone in a twin bed with a firm mattress. I missed snuggling with Kal, but we both rested better in separate beds. I was up and down frequently during the night, and often found myself awake at odd hours, reading or watching TV. When watching television, I adopted a half-seated position with a pillow under my knees to reduce pressure on the incision, which I greatly desired.

Sitting fully upright was difficult for some time. Kal had a recliner chair, which I adjusted in a partially leaned-back position. I was often more comfortable in the recliner than lying in bed. I could adjust the chair periodically to alter my weight distribution, and it was a lot easier to get up from a semi-seated position than lying down.

~ ~

At the dinner table, I sat with a pillow under me; even so, fifteen minutes was about my limit. Besides getting tired, I would develop a headache. It took ten days or so to get over the headaches and get so I could sit up longer. I quickly learned not to push it — when my body told me to stop whatever I was doing, I obeyed.

Standing up for periods of time was impossible at first and difficult for many weeks following the surgery. When I found myself tiring, I simply had to find somewhere to sit or lie down. When walking, it was with short steps rather than my usual long-strided gait. After several days I realized I walked stooped-over forward. I had adjusted instinctively to my physical condition, bending in the middle to keep from stretching the abdomen. I gradually straightened up as I felt stronger, but it was at least two months after the surgery before I returned to good posture. And then, after weeks of slumping, I had to keep reminding myself to stand up straight.

I also found it was difficult to sustain a conversation for any length of time. I tired very quickly and I had trouble concentrating for very long. So I stopped trying, and would go off to read or take another nap.

By the time I left the hospital I had returned to a normal diet, although I was not up to eating anything spicy, heavy or fatty. I concentrated on low-fat foods that were easy to fix and digest — yogurt, cereal, fruit, soup, pasta, fish and chicken were staples. Although I drank prune juice daily to offset the side effects of the pain medications and antibiotics, I experienced considerable gas, flatulation and constipation for many weeks. I also stayed away from alcohol long after I was off the various drugs; I was still shaky, and drinking simply had no appeal.

Five days after the operation, I started taking the synthetic hormones, a drug I knew I would be living with for many years. I waited five days because my body was so upset I figured it did not need any more problems. By then I was having hot flashes. Apparently, it took my body that long to deplete the estrogen stored in my fat cells and react to the fact that my ovaries, and my supply of natural hormones, were gone. (Heavier women actually have a slight advantage at this point, since estrogen is stockpiled in fatty tissues. More fat cells means more estrogen, although that formula certainly should not be carried too far.) As I swallowed the first pill, I studied the list of possible side affects. It was daunting: headaches, dizziness, leg pains, chest pains, nausea, bloating, yellowing of the eyes or skin, mental changes. Fortunately, I never exhibited any of the numerous problems, although a category as vague as "mental changes" leaves a lot of room.

ABOUT HORMONE REPLACEMENT THERAPY

Hormone replacement therapy (HRT) is the use of synthetic hormones to supplement or replace those produced naturally by a woman's ovaries. Hormone production stops gradually as a part of menopause or instantly when the ovaries are removed surgically. Whether synthetic hormones should be employed is a matter of considerable controversy, both within the medical and lay communities. The issue is one of great significance to women because hormones affect every aspect of a woman's life, health and well-being. Estrogen is especially important; it is known to signifi-

cantly lower a woman's risk of developing both heart disease and osteoporosis, the brittle bone disease, and may lower the risks of colon cancer and dying of Alzheimer's disease. Estrogen has also been referred to as a virtual elixir of youth for women. By slowing the ravages of time, it forestalls hot flashes, night sweats, vaginal dryness and other miseries of menopause, improves mental functioning and concentration and helps preserve skin elasticity and color. The influence of estrogen on sexual desire and performance is even more basic. Without this hormone, the vagina returns to its prepubescent shape (narrow, shorter, less elastic) and condition (drier). Sex may become painful or less pleasurable and the libido may simply disappear.

Among women who undergo oophorectomy, the matter of HRT is fairly clear-cut. Removal of the ovaries before natural menopause produces an instant, dramatic and potentially devastating plunge into menopause, with resulting hot flashes, depression, diminished sexual function, loss of mental acuity and a variety of other menopausal symptoms. Synthetic estrogen counteracts the loss of the ovaries, reducing menopausal symptoms and producing the desired protection against heart and bone disease. However, treatment must continue indefinitely, which could mean taking estrogen for years or even decades.

Women who have a hysterectomy but keep their ovaries will continue to produce natural estrogen and progesterone until menopause occurs. At that time, these women must decide on HRT based on the merits of treatment relative to their personal situations and desires.

For women who undergo natural, non-surgical menopause, the HRT issue can be extremely problematic.

When in the natural menopause sequence to start HRT, in what dosages, how often and for how long, are all unresolved issues, as is the link to cancer, high blood pressure, diabetes and other conditions. Side effects vary, on both the plus and minus sides. Many women report feeling more like themselves, with more energy, better concentration and improved short-term memory. Recent studies also indicate HRT can improve stress incontinence, relieve vaginal dryness and may decrease the risk of Alzheimer's disease. On the negative side are irregular bleeding for women who still have periods, mood swings and irritability, breast tenderness, bloating, acne, depression, cramping and headaches, most of which are related to the progesterone portion of the cycle. On the cautionary front, one piece of recent research appears to show a relationship between long-term use of estrogen and increased risk of breast cancer and other malignancies. Another study found no correlation between increased risk of cancer and HRT.

Among many in medical circles, support for HRT is strong, especially since the average female life expectancy is now 78 years of age. That means women face many years (the average age at time of menopause is the early 50s) in which they are vulnerable to heart disease, osteoporosis and other conditions related to estrogen deficiency. Supporters of HRT believe the benefits of long-term treatment outweigh the possible risks, making estrogen America's number one selling drug.

~ ~

Skeptics are equally vocal, accusing proponents of HRT of being mostly male and/or medical professionals who are biased toward excessive dependence on drugs, and generally out of touch with the needs of women. They suggest natural relief of menopausal symptoms, especially hot flashes, lies in proper diet, exercise, avoiding excessive drinking and not smoking. To guard against osteoporosis, many advise women to take daily calcium supplements and to eat generous supplies of dairy products, fish and dark green vegetables.

Even more fundamental is the debate about life phases. Many women, backed by medical professionals, prefer to let nature take its course. They learn to enjoy the new life stages reached after natural cessation of estrogen production, rather than treating menopause as a disease that requires decades of medication. Other women, also supported by medical opinion, see no reason to give in to the aging process. A hundred years ago, women often did not outlive the production of their ovaries. Now, as women lead longer lives, the entire issue of HRT becomes increasingly urgent and complex.

The fact is, less than 30 percent of American women practice HRT on a long-term basis. Many begin therapy and quit after a year or two, often because of irregular bleeding. Expense is another factor, especially among women who do not have insurance coverage adequate to cover the average $30-per-month cost.

As with so many matters surrounding women's health, HRT is not well-researched, and there are no clear-cut answers. In making a decision, each woman

must access her personal situation, medical history
and values, and ask her doctor to lay out the risks,
benefits and unknowns. Then she must decide for
herself.

UH OH, IS THIS A PROBLEM?

Ten days after the surgery I was definitely feeling
stronger — sleeping less, sitting up and conversing for
extended periods, even sitting outside briefly for a breath of
fresh air.

Part of my bedtime routine was changing my sanitary
napkin; as expected, I had had a discharge since the surgery,
typically brownish and fairly light.

Not this time. Suddenly the pad was saturated and
bright red.

Was something wrong? Why was I bleeding? Should I
call the doctor? I decided to wait until morning and see what
happened.

Morning brought more blood. I called Dr. Finn as
soon as her office opened. She told me to come in. I was not
driving yet and Kal had left for work so I called my
daughter. The ride to the doctor's office was my first since
the operation; those Michigan potholes once again had my
name all over them, but I adjusted the seat back and endured
the trip.

Dr. Finn checked me both internally and externally.
She found some bleeding high up inside the vagina, in the
area where my uterus had been attached. As it turned out,
the problem was not serious — just some stitches that had

weakened. A quick and painless cauterizing ended the bleeding, which, as she explained, was fairly common at this stage post-surgery. Still, the experience was unsettling, because bleeding was a complication I knew could be dangerous.

By the time my daughter drove me back to Kal's, I was completely exhausted. I spent that afternoon taking a long nap.

There were a couple other outings in those first two weeks after surgery, one a brief sojourn to a wedding shower and the other to take care of some family business. In each case my daughter provided the transportation; both times I returned completely drained from the effort and ended up spending the next day in bed.

Mostly I was well behaved during the first weeks after surgery; I followed instructions and did not try to do more than I was supposed to. The truth was, I could not. My body simply would not allow me to do anything other than let itself heal.

THERE'S ONLY ONE THING TO DO AFTER HYSTERECTOMY

For the first weeks after surgery, rest and recuperation is all a woman can, or should, try to do. Because no matter what type of surgical procedure is employed, having an operation of the magnitude of a hysterectomy represents a tremendous insult to the body. It is a serious injury, albeit an intentional, controlled and skillfully performed one, and recovering from any injury takes time.

Fortunately, medical science has learned a great deal in recent years about how to encourage the body to recover.

When my mother had surgery, in 1971, her feet did not touch the floor for three full days. She was allowed only to stand up for another day or two after that; then, finally, she actually started walking. By then, the lack of muscular and heart activity had exacerbated the weakness caused by the actual operation. So she was fighting back on two fronts. Her hospitalization lasted a week, which was a typical hospital stay for hysterectomy two and a half decades ago. (Mom had a vertical incision, running from just below the navel to just above the pubic hair. The bikini-style cut that is now typical came into general use later. In addition to being more aesthetically pleasing for the patient, the horizontal cut is less subject to stress and injury than the older, vertical incision. But medical people say a vertical cut is still used in emergency situations, because it is easier to perform and affords the doctor a better view of what is going on inside the patient.)

In contrast to my mom's experience, I was up the very night that I had my operation, as I have mentioned, and walking by the next day, although protesting vigorously all the way. Dr. Finn had ordered me to be up and around and active, within the very real limits of someone who had just had her insides cut open. "The human heart is designed to beat against gravity," she pointed out. "Lying down all the time does you more harm than good. I want you to get up out of bed in the morning, and sit up for periods of time during the day, to make your heart work like it's supposed to. That will help you feel better faster than staying in bed." These days, after a hysterectomy, women are almost always on their feet and walking in less than twenty-four hours.

~ ~ ~ ~ ~ ~ ~ ~ ~ ~ ~ ~ ~ ~ ~ ~ ~ ~ ~ ~

That does not mean we may be comfortable doing it. "I knew intellectually that I had to get up," remembered Helen, one of the women who shared her experience with me. "But my body said no, no, no."

The plain truth is, pain goes with the territory, as do grogginess, wooziness, nausea, loss of appetite and generally feeling really bad.

"Majorly uncomfortable," continued Helen, describing how she felt in the initial post-surgery period. "I wanted more pain medication: I practically begged the nurse. But she couldn't give me a larger dose without an order from the doctor, which we finally got. The down-side of getting more is that pain medication dopes you up pretty good, when you're already out of it from the anesthesia and the trauma. It takes at least two weeks for all that stuff to completely metabolize out of the system." Helen, as mentioned previously, heads a women's hospital unit, so she speaks from experience about such things. In recalling the first week or so after surgery, she concluded, "You just feel so awful. You expect to feel better, but you really don't for a while."

The variations in treatment for post-surgery pain are, once again, considerable. Some physicians prescribe a pain pump, such as the one I had. Others use various combinations of injections and, in one case, exterior support.

Lea's doctor put a tight elastic-type binder around her abdomen, which he kept in place for two weeks after surgery. "I wasn't all that sore," she remembered. "I believe the binder really helped."

Some women try to ignore their discomfort, like Victoria, who described herself as learning to play over the pain in sports and doing the same with her hysterectomy. Or

~ ~

Alice, who took herself off pain pills after three days because she did not like the sensation that "the stuff was attacking my brain as well as my incision." Absent serious complications, most women taper off medications within ten days after surgery, as their pain subsides.

Women who have the vaginal procedure, with no abdominal incision, get off pain killers a bit sooner, although they still experience major discomfort inside. (In some recent cases following uncomplicated vaginal hysterectomy, hospitals are actually discharging patients the day of surgery, at the insistence of insurance companies seeking to cut costs. Reaction is mixed, with many doctors and patients feeling the practice puts women at risk.)

Just as it involves pain, there is no way around the fact that a hysterectomy puts a woman out of commission with substantial disability during the first two or three weeks. Planning ahead to arrange some type of assistance at home, whether having a relative or friend come in to help with children and housework, or sending the kids to stay else-where, is a necessity. After the surgery, we require, and deserve, all the help we can get.

That is not always an easy thing for us to do. Women are used to being the people who get things done. Jody spoke for many of us when she said:

"All I wanted to do for those first two weeks was lie down. I had absolutely no energy, and that was very disturbing to me. I felt guilty. I actually found myself apologizing to people when I had to let them do things for me."

I had similar feelings, especially when Kal had to make late-night trips to the grocery or run to the 24-hour pharmacy at six in the morning before starting his own

~ ~

hectic day. I learned to let him do it, though, because I had no other choice.

Luckily for most of us, and for our families, immediate post-hysterectomy complications are relatively minor — a stitch that does not heal, an infection of some kind, an itchy incision, prolonged drainage. Very harsh gas and severe constipation are also very common. In fact, every woman I talked to experienced such problems. As one nurse put it, "I'll never, ever make light of a patient who complains of gas again. Now I know how bad it can be."

Loss of appetite is typical, too, although Lynn was the rare exception who said she was "real hungry" right after surgery. Most of us have to wait a couple of weeks before regaining much interest in food.

Still, any woman facing a hysterectomy needs to be aware the surgery can carry real risk, as Gail's experience illustrates so well.

"I had a vaginal hysterectomy, actually a long time ago, in 1971. About ten days after the surgery, I hemorrhaged. I was gushing blood. We stuffed towels between my legs as my husband drove me to the hospital. The towels turned bright red. When we got there, I was rushed into intensive care; I had transfusions going into both arms. I almost died; I lost eight pints of blood before they finally got it stopped. We found out later that because I had a vaginal procedure, and the surgeon couldn't see what he was doing, he didn't use enough stitches inside of me. And the ones that were there dissolved before I was healed. That's when I hemorrhaged. I guess we should have sued for malpractice, but I was just so grateful to be alive. The doctor stopped practicing soon after this happened, whether because of my brush with death, I don't know."

Then, sometimes, there's also a lighter side to be found in the midst of discomfort. Lea remembered:

"The day of my operation was also the day Lorena Bobbitt did her special brand of surgery on her husband. My husband read to me how she cut off her husband's penis while he was sleeping, when he came home drunk after being with another woman. The newspapers and magazines made every comment imaginable, and a lot of it was very amusing, and suggestive. It hurt so much to laugh, but I laughed anyhow. I couldn't help it, it was just so funny."

Individual variations in experience aside, Alice's description of how she felt in the first two weeks after surgery was typical of my experience and that of most women after a hysterectomy: "I was just plain out of it."

❧

WHAT WAS IMPORTANT

Based on my experience, more learning and words of advice.

1. Don't try to do anything. Just negotiating the basics, like eating, getting in and out of bed and going to the bathroom, is absolutely all you can expect to do.

2. Concentrate on what you need to do to recu- perate. Like many women, my hectic schedule

~ ~ ~ ~ ~ ~ ~ ~ ~ ~ ~ ~ ~ ~ ~ ~ ~ ~ ~ ~

often left little time for taking care of myself. I spent those first post-surgery days doing nothing but that — reading, sleeping, watching television, sitting, phoning and generally minimizing any distractions.

3. Ask for help. Obviously, in the hospital, that was necessary, but the same was true after coming home. I could not run out to the supermarket or the drug store; somebody had to do all those things for me. So, I let others do things, and gladly accepted their aid.

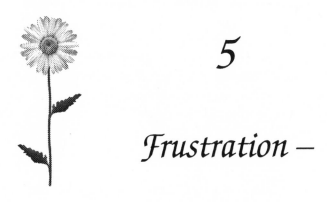

5

Frustration –

Three To Five Weeks

~ ~

A Friday evening in mid-May, with the pleasant softness of high spring blowing gently through the open window, carrying in the freshness of budding trees and the scent of flowers eager for another day.

I sat on the couch in my family room, feet tucked up beside me, a bunched-up pillow supporting my back. As I hung up the phone, I sagged back into the cushions.

"Damn, I hate this!" The cat, snuggled next to me, turned to check the source of the disturbance. "That's the second invitation I've turned down tonight!"

The first was a long-planned excursion to help my friend Ann open her cottage for the summer. The cottage, for many years one of my very favorite places, had been the scene of my bloody Memorial Day weekend in 1991 and

~ ~

my recuperation after the endometrial ablation in 1992. The location was an easy hour's drive from home, so close we could make it for dinner after a full day's work.

But not this Friday. When Ann called to verify the time of our departure, I had to cancel — I was absolutely, completely exhausted; I just could not go.

Within a half hour another friend called with a last-minute ticket to a local advertising function. I turned that down, too.

Then I cried — because I had no energy, because I wanted to do what I wanted to do, because I was worried by my unaccustomed weariness, because I wanted to feel better and get back to normal and because I was not there yet.

RECUPERATION VARIATIONS

Where and how we recover from hysterectomy can vary widely, depending on individual needs and circumstances, and the type and extent of surgery.

Doctors generally cite six weeks as the minimum period of time required to recuperate. Typically, women go home after being released from the hospital, and depend on assistance from family and friends. I went back and forth between my house and Kal's, spending the first two weeks at his place, then a week at my house, then back to his and finally home for good, a month after my surgery.

Although most of us resume normal activities like driving, cleaning and light cooking two to three weeks after surgery, gradually adding more tasks after that, the best description of what happens after a hysterectomy was provided by Trudy, who said, "You may look okay, which

~ ~ ~ ~ ~ ~ ~ ~ ~ ~ ~ ~ ~ ~ ~ ~ ~ ~ ~ ~

means people expect you to act okay. But you sure aren't recovered from a hysterectomy in two or three weeks."

Actually, some women bounced back fairly quickly, like Donna, who said she was cooking easy dinners for her family two weeks after surgery.

My mom was doing light housework after three. (Vacuuming, by the way, is universally regarded as an absolute restriction for at least six weeks. Apparently the repetitive back-and forth motion pulls on injured internal tissues, causing damage. No great loss; I never liked vacuuming and I do not know many women who do.)

Jody's ex-husband took their five children to his house for five weeks, which gave her a chance to recover in peace and quiet. She described this interval as "the longest vacation I'll ever have."

Other women found their vacation cottages the ideal place to regain their strength. Like Mary:

"My daughter drove me to our place on the lake two weeks after my operation. I just sat there on the deck and took it easy. Looking out over that water was a real tonic for me."

Lynn approached recovery very aggressively:

"Like most things, it became a competition for me. I started on the exercise bike a week after the surgery. I was on the stepper in two weeks, and the Nordic Trak at three. Abdominal workouts came at three and a half weeks — my doctor knew me well enough to agree to all this. It was me against the illness; my recovery was a competition to do better."

Trudy, who was a teacher at the time of her surgery, had timed the operation so she would have the entire summer to recuperate. "I got permission to gradually add

~ ~

activities," she remembered. "I liked having visitors, especially after I started feeling strong enough to get stir crazy. I also did sit-down activities, like cleaning my button box."

She also remembered an important truth about the recovery period. "I got so terribly, unbelievably tired. I just had no reserves."

BLAM! DAMN! SHUTDOWN!

Three weeks after surgery, I was certainly feeling better. Some semblance of normal activity had returned — driving, grocery shopping (I did ask for help carrying out the bags the first couple of times), cooking, meeting with friends. All that was encouraging, feeling like I could do the familiar things that make up everyday life.

I also got acquainted with what became, for me, the most frustrating aspect of the entire hysterectomy process, something I came to call "The Shutdown."

My doctor had warned me that I would get unbelievably tired during recovery. But I was completely unprepared for the totality of The Shutdown. It was in complete contrast to my usual mind-over-matter strategy for negotiating a hectic schedule — no matter how tired I got, I could always somehow find enough energy to carry on.

Until I had the hysterectomy.

When The Shutdown hit, my body just stopped. It absolutely refused to go any further. No amount of self-talk — "Come on, Sue, you can do it," "Just a little bit longer, then you can rest," "Get going, you wimp!" — improved things as The Shutdown took over. At those times I was utterly depleted. For the first time in my life, I simply could not go on.

Instead of mind over matter, I was confronted with matter over mind — suddenly my unobeying body completely and irrevocably took over, demanding that I cease whatever I was doing and go to bed.

This was completely new territory for me. After all, I was a woman who indulged in such challenges as cross-country skiing 30 kilometer races over uphill terrain in zero degree weather, riding a bicycle 75 miles into a head wind so fierce it was tough to stay upright, and working 30 hours straight when a tight deadline demanded. Suddenly, I could not drag myself through the most mundane sort of day.

The Shutdown was blinding, mind-numbing fatigue. I learned to feel it coming, first as a sort of generalized weariness, progressing gradually until it spread over me like a haze. I could not deal with anybody or anything when under the influence of The Shutdown. I was irritable and short-tempered, even with Kal and my children and my closest friends. I did not want to eat because it took too much effort. I could not read because it was too demanding. I could not think logically and rationally about anything other than resting — immediately!

Accompanying The Shutdown was a phenomenon known as a "flat affect." I felt little or no sense of the multi-dimensional animation that surrounds a healthy person; my body and personality were compressed into a single deflated dimension — vague, lackluster and dull.

In the early stages of recovery, I dropped into a quick sleep during The Shutdown. Later, I found that merely "stretching" — getting off my feet to lie down and rest — allowed me to rejuvenate enough to carry on. On those occasions when I was able to get myself through a task, I paid for it by spending the next day or two exhausted, close to home and bed.

Driving was especially taxing. Getting in and out of the car required care and effort, and actually piloting a vehicle required a level of attention and awareness that was difficult to maintain. On several occasions I was driving when I probably was not fit to do so. At those times, my only thought was to get wherever I was going so I could collapse.

THE GREAT UNIVERSAL — FATIGUE

If there was one aspect of post-hysterectomy recuperation that everyone seemed to agree on, this was it.

Incredible fatigue.

"I got tired so easily," was how Lea put it.

"Stamina was the real challenge," recalled Sheryl.

"I didn't anticipate the exhaustion," was Jody's comment. "I'm still amazed at how tired I was. It scared me."

Whether in remarks from the women I talked to, or published commentary in magazines and books, extended post-surgical tiredness was a common denominator. Even women who came into surgery healthy (except for the symptoms that got them there) and convinced a hysterectomy was necessary, said it took them at least six weeks to feel like they had any type of energy again.

Sheryl remembered, "I'd start to walk across the room, and I'd get overwhelmed with fatigue. I actually had to sit down on the floor to keep from just crumpling down in a heap."

~ ~

That is an experience I can certainly relate to. Because while I never physically collapsed, I frequently grabbed onto tables, chair backs, counter tops, car doors, Kal, my children and any other sturdy object that was available for support. And I did that for many weeks.

"It took me quite a while to feel good again," was Helen's assessment of her situation. "As a nurse, I could understand the medical explanation — all the body's energy was going into healing, which left nothing for anything else. I found there were a lot of little plateaus — like sleeping through the night was a real accomplishment — but it seemed like it took a long while to get to the next one. I really expected to feel better much sooner than I did."

Lynn, for whom recovery was a competition, described fatigue as her only real complication. "I'd walk down to the barn and it felt like a ten-mile run."

Even the most welcome activities could become an effort. Mary talked about the visit of a friend. "We walked from the house down to the river and back, which normally I do without even thinking. I was absolutely exhausted! I couldn't wait for her to leave so I could go to sleep."

SECOND GUESSING

Physically, my overt symptoms continued to improve rapidly. The incision was healing nicely, I was beginning to walk more normally and color was returning to my cheeks.

So why was I so tired? Why could I not carry on in a normal manner? Frustrated, I wondered if I were imagining the fatigue I was feeling. Surely the inability to get through even the simplest of days was all in my head.

~ ~

Often during this time, I found myself questioning the wisdom of my decision to have a hysterectomy — I had been duped by the medical establishment after all — the bleeding hadn't been as bad as I thought — the problem would have gone away by itself eventually — I should have waited out menopause.

Oh, God, I fretted, had I made a horrible, irreversible mistake?

I knew that many women experience depression after a hysterectomy. But I did not feel depressed — I felt frustrated!

So I talked to my sister. I called Dr. Finn. I wanted to know why I was still so tired. I wanted to understand why it was taking me so long to feel decent. I wanted reassurance that I had not been taken advantage of. I wanted to know I had made the right choice.

Both assured me that my physical symptoms and feelings of frustration were normal. Major surgery, my sister explained to me, insults the body enough to require a period of recuperation. Fatigue was in reaction to this trauma, a clear demand that the body be given the time it needs to recover. She advised me that healing of the internal tissues takes a minimum of eight weeks.

Dr. Finn, after listening sympathetically to my fatigue-induced fretting, reminded me that I was probably more impatient at the pace of recovery than a women accustomed to a less hectic schedule. She also indicated that my body would progress at its own pace and there was little I could do about it but wait. In fact, she cautioned, trying to hurry things too fast could actually result in prolonging the recuperation. Patience was the necessary order of the day.

~ ~

Patience had never been one of my virtues, but I tried to find some. Meanwhile, I called Dr. Finn's office again. This time I talked to her nurse. "Doctor is very conservative and would not even consider doing surgery unless she was convinced it was the best thing for you," the nurse assured me. Later, Dr. Finn said the same thing.

"I have never and would not ever perform a hysterectomy or any other surgery that I did not believe was completely medically justified and in the best interests of my patient.

"The decision to have a hysterectomy is so individualized. I can provide the medical perspective, but each woman must make her own decision, based on her own circumstances. Most hysterectomies are done, as you know, to improve quality of life. Ultimately, the only person who can decide how much her life is being compromised, and how having a hysterectomy may improve it, is you."

So I waited, trying to listen to my body and respond to what it was telling me I could and could not do. I wanted to feel better; I expected to feel better. Part of the problem was, I did not know how much "better" I was supposed to feel.

Gradually, the time between my shutdowns did lengthen, and my energy began to return. But I continued to get stopped short by the impenetrable barrier of tiredness off and on for several months. Meanwhile, surrounding me was a houseful of long-delayed projects, and I lamented the fact that at last, when I finally had time to tackle them, I lacked the energy to get anything done.

MORE POST-SURGERY SYMPTOMS

There were a number of other tangible reminders during these weeks of what had happened to me.

Although the incision was largely healed, I experienced heaviness and tightness in my abdomen. My gut felt like I was carrying a watermelon around inside it; the skin was pulled and distended and hard. The inch or so immediately surrounding the cut was numb to the touch and rigid. Occasionally, even after the real pain had subsided, I would have sudden twinges flash through my midsection, not pain so much as a fleeting sting.

My cat did not help. She was delighted to have me around so much, and she proved it by snuggling close and purring every chance she got. But her settling down invariably included a walk across my stomach. "Ow, ow, ow!" I grimaced as her feet, one by pointed one, dug into me. But I enjoyed having her keep me company.

There were other changes as well, several of them mental. I found my thinking processes were not as acute as I was used to them being. I had trouble putting thoughts together; making even simple decisions was frequently a chore. I also experienced nightmares and had trouble sleeping, awakening after a few hours sleep unable to doze back off. I still remember dreaming my younger grandson had died, and no one told me for three days because they did not want to upset me. I awoke from that one in a panic and short of breath. Often during those weeks I was irritable and short-tempered, especially in the midst of a shutdown. I found the top of my left hand was sore to the touch. And I had a lot of frequent, often harsh, gas.

~ ~

Dr. Finn assured me all my symptoms were well within the normal reaction to surgery. The numbness around my incision was the result of the nerves, skin, muscles and other tissue being separated. The heaviness and the twinges would disappear gradually, although she said I would probably have such episodes for many years and possibly the rest of my life. Disturbances in thinking patterns and sleeping, with the attendant difficulty in making decisions and having nightmares, frequently were the after-effects of general anesthesia and the attendant disruption of normal mental functioning. The soreness in my hand was from the intravenous needle that was inserted into a vein at that location. The gas was caused by the reluctance of my intestinal track to return to normal.

The severity of some of my post-hysterectomy symptoms, especially the sleep disturbances, mental vagueness and the roller coaster fatigue, were exacerbated by the removal of my ovaries. These are all common side effects of menopause; the decrease in estrogen levels and the abruptness of my alternation heightened the symptoms. Even though I had started taking hormone pills after the surgery, what had happened to my system was not a natural withdrawal. It took a while to adjust to its new circumstances. Meanwhile, my symptoms were reminders my body was not entirely happy about its new condition

INFORMATION, PLEASE

It was during this time frame that I became aware of the dearth of solid, detailed information on what a woman might expect to experience following a hysterectomy. I checked the bookstore and found several generalized

~ ~

volumes on women's health that included hysterectomy as a chapter, and a few books on hysterectomy per se. But current treatment of the subject was largely accusatory — decrying the number of hysterectomies performed and labeling a substantial percentage as unnecessary. Obviously that did not do me any good — I had already made my decision and was looking for more on the aftermath.

I did a search of recent periodicals with much the same result.

I was left to wonder and worry on my own: was what I was feeling normal for two weeks, three weeks, five weeks following the operation? Was my pace of recovery on target? What about all the twitches, twinges, hesitations, pangs, pricks, itches, tingles and yes, improvements, I was experiencing? How was I supposed to deal with all that had been happening to me? Was I reacting normally? What and when was I supposed to think and do and feel?

I worried that I was being a nuisance with repeated calls to my doctor and my sister. I feared that my questions were stupid. I imagined that I had become hopelessly neurotic. I concluded that I had descended into hypochondria. The professionals all assured me that my responses and frustrations were perfectly normal and urged me to continue to ask any and all questions about my condition.

I quickly concluded that what I was really needed was detail, and lots of it, about every aspect of surgery and recovery, from someone who had been there, through the entire experience, beginning to end.

I reasoned that if I was disconcerted by the lack of information, other women must be making the same search, with the same unsatisfactory results. So I started keeping track of the progress of my recovery, writing down the details and minutia I could not find anywhere else. This volume is the result.

ACHOO!

I never thought that a simple sneeze could be a major milestone. Yet I remember this particular sneeze clearly, because it was a dramatic demonstration that something was not only different, it was better!

One morning, as I was walking into the bathroom, something tickled my nose. So I sneezed, hard. I had gotten beyond the gut-grabbing phase of recovery, so I did not think much of it for the first moment or two.

Then something monumental dawned on me — I did not leak! For the first time in as long as I could remember, I sneezed and did not end up with a wet spot on my underwear!

"Yes!" I shouted out loud. "All right!" I rejoiced with the image in the mirror. "I'll be damned," I laughed. "The bladder suspension worked, it really worked!"

Later, I shared the news with Kal, although I doubt that someone who had not spent years afraid to cough suddenly or laugh with gusto could fully appreciate the significance of this historic occasion.

More important was the meaning of this moment for me: after months of agonizing over the decision to have surgery, after four weeks of pain and discomfort, after difficult moments of self-doubt and second-guessing, this was tangible confirmation that my decision to have surgery was an appropriate one. My life really was going to be improved as a result.

MORE NORMAL STUFF

Gradually, as my stamina increased, I was able to pick up my level of activity. Typically, I might be able to carry out one out-of-home activity per day, although I still required rest time, and The Shutdown always loomed.

Kal and I began to resume some affectionate sex play, but we faithfully adhered to the no-penetration admonition for the requisite eight weeks. Nevertheless, it was good for me to know that I could still get turned on, that all the messing around with my female apparatus and the advent of synthetic hormones had not snuffed out my sex drive.

I made my first foray into a social setting four weeks after the operation, to an engagement party for friends of my son. I took my camera and managed to get some good photos. I also tried drinking alcohol for the first time. Even though I had been off all medications for at least two weeks, a few tentative sips of beer made me light-headed and woozy. I stopped drinking and did not try it again for another week. After about ninety minutes of socializing, I drove home and promptly went to bed.

The next afternoon, a Sunday, I skipped church but went to the opera; one big activity per day was still all I could manage. Ann picked me up at home, drove us to the theater, dropped me off and picked me up at the door to minimize my walking, and we enjoyed the show. But I was in bed by 8:30 that evening, more than ready to get off my feet.

Four and a half weeks after the surgery I attended a wedding with the permission of both my gynecologist and my urologist. But no dancing, they warned. Just sit and watch. I did, except when the bride threw her bouquet. I

~ ~

lined up with the other single women — there were about fifteen of us ranging in age from college kids to those who were considerably older. Right at me! "I hope you didn't jump," Dr. Finn said when I told her about it. Nope; in fact, I had to put my hands up to keep the flowers from hitting me in the head.

All these incidents were small in the normal scope of things, but the parties and the opera were important as indicators that I was getting back to normal. "Little celebrations," were what one woman called them. They let me know I could once again enjoy the company of others and do the sorts of things I expected to be able to do.

WHAT WAS IN THERE

Both Dr. Finn and Dr. Andrews pronounced my recuperation "on track" during post-surgery appointments. I went in to their offices with my usual lists of questions, looking for more detailed information about the recovery process and what was and might not be normal at this stage of things.

Dr. Finn had received my pathology report — analysis of uterine, tubal and ovarian tissue is always done following surgery. All my tests were negative for any cancerous conditions; what a relief! I also learned that my uterus had weighed nearly a pound and a half; a normal uterus weighs about three ounces. I had more than twenty fibroid masses, and they were everywhere; inside the uterus, outside the organ, and embedded in the muscular wall. Individually, the fibroids were not exceptionally large, with sizes ranging from less than an inch to about three inches. But because there were so many of them, my entire abdominal cavity was involved. My uterus had gotten so large that it had run out of room to grow in normal areas, and had worked into the cul-de-sac area behind my bladder, adding pressure there.

Analysis of my ovaries and tubes showed the right side was normal in size and appearance. The left ovary was enlarged to more than twice the size it should have been, with a blood-filled cyst on the surface. The left tube was dilated, more than twice the normal length and width, and filled with fluid. There was also considerable endometriosis throughout my abdominal cavity, and adhesions fusing my various tissues together.

What that all added up to was a lot more of a mess than Dr. Finn had been able to anticipate before she got inside to take a good look. Despite all that, my blood loss during surgery had been minimal, about half a pint.

We reviewed my hormone status; because I was having hot flashes, Dr. Finn increased the dosage and ordered a blood test to measure my hormone levels. My last task was to collect a letter for my employer, stating that I was fit to go to work.

BACK TO WORK — SORT OF

Returning to work was the next big hurdle, which I did five weeks following the surgery. In reality, I was dabbling with returning to work, showing up just long enough to get paid. My doctors would have preferred a six-week break, but my medical leave dropped from full to half-pay at five weeks, and I could not afford to take the financial hit. Still, I was more fortunate than many women, to have as much paid leave as I did.

~ ~

That first morning back was a real revelation; for one thing, I had never paid much attention to how much effort it takes just to get up, get ready and drive to the office.

The welcome back was warm and encouraging, accompanied by exclamations that I had lost a lot of weight. Actually, my surgery-related loss was only five pounds or so, but I retained enough gauntness and pallor to make me look thinner than I actually was.

Several of my female co-workers got a little gift that morning. I had collected all my tampons and carefully wrapped them in festive paper with colorful ribbons. The card that went with each present said, "Just for you! A little something I won't be needing anymore." Every one of the women knew what was in the package without even opening it. One of my friends still keeps her unopened gift on a shelf in her office. "When I need a good laugh, I look at it," she says. "It really helps lighten up a bad day."

I made it that first day until 2 o'clock. By noon I could feel The Shutdown crawling up over me. When I finally left the office, it was all I could do to drive myself home. Blindly tired, I stumbled upstairs and fell into bed, too far into the stupor to remove my clothes. I slept until 8:00 that evening, got up long enough to find something to eat, and was back in bed by 9:15.

The next day I lasted until 3 o'clock, then went home and surrendered myself to The Shutdown for the remainder of the day. Fortunately, my first two days at the office were on Thursday and Friday, which gave me the weekend to recuperate. I knew I was a long way from being back to normal, and that I was going to need all the strength I could find to negotiate an entire week of work.

TAKE THAT JOB ... AND LOVE IT?

While getting back to work is an important indicator of health and vitality after a hysterectomy, it can also be, as it was for me, a taxing and tiring step.

Although I, and most of the women I interviewed, are employed, women who are engaged in the business of taking care of home and family full-time face the same sort of challenge. In that case, the return to activity may be more gradual, rather that the abrupt today-you-go-back-to-work that I faced. The temptation for women whose work is at home may be to do too much too soon, especially when there are young children who demand attention.

No matter what our job, or where we do it, getting back after a hysterectomy takes grit and determination.

Lynn beat most women by returning to her career as managing physician of a busy emergency room just three and a half weeks after her operation. Going back that soon was not entirely a matter of choice, said Lynn, who added she would have been a happy woman if she could have taken the normal six weeks off:

"We were terribly shorthanded, and my other doctors had been pulling extra shifts to cover for me while I was out. Besides, the way we're set up, if we don't work we don't get paid, so that was additional motivation. Work was really tough, especially because I'm on my feet constantly, running from patient to patient. I'd get so tired I'd break out in a sweat — I felt like I had the flu. When that happened, I'd go rest for a while. That fixed me up enough to get through a shift."

~ ~ ~ ~ ~ ~ ~ ~ ~ ~ ~ ~ ~ ~ ~ ~ ~ ~ ~ ~

Mary went back to her job with the state government after five weeks, although she worked half-days for the first two weeks. She remembered, "I was tired at first, but those half days let me ease back in."

Lea resumed teaching six weeks to the day after her surgery. Helen also went back to the nursing unit she heads after six weeks. "I can't imagine going back any sooner," she said. "Five weeks would have just been too early. The problem," she continued, "is that our system of work and society doesn't allow us enough time to really recover. It takes at least eight weeks after a hysterectomy to feel decent and energetic again."

Just because we look halfway decent does not mean we are back to 100 percent.

❧

WHAT WAS IMPORTANT

What I learned at this point in the process.

1. Plan on an extended recovery period. There is no way around the fact it is going to take at least six weeks to resume a semblance of normal functioning.

2. Be patient! Recovery takes a long time, much longer than I had anticipated, and all I could do was wait.

3. Increase activities gradually. Much as I would have liked to plunge right back into a full schedule, I was not able to do so. Instead, I had to take it slow and add tasks carefully; other-

~ ~

wise, I overextended my capabilities and ended up paying for it.

4. Listen to your body. Although my doctors had warned me I would have to take it easy, it was my body that finally got me to pay attention. It spoke loudly, and when it told me to stop and rest, that is exactly what I had to do.

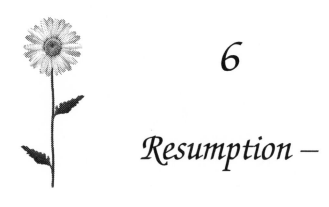

6

Resumption –

Six To Eight Weeks

~ ~

I saw myself riding in a bus, a stripped-down school transportation model, minding my own business, looking out the window at woodsy scenery going by. Out of the corner of my eye I noticed a man walking past me down the aisle. He paused beside my seat and set a box next to me. Strange, I thought. What could be in this carton and why would the guy put it here.

The bus bumped along for a few minutes, the bouncing gradually jarring loose the lid of the box. I became aware of something poking out of the container and reaching toward me.

A snake!

Then another, both heads extended in my direction, swaying slightly as the bus sped along. Startled, I gasped

~ ~

and shrank back against the window. There was no place to go — the snakes blocked my exit and I could not get away.

They kept staring at me, apparently not interested in making an attack. Gradually, I realized that their eyes were not hostile, as I might have expected, but quizzical. They continued their movement toward me. I relaxed slightly; although wary of snakes, I was not terrified by these two. Finally, both of the creatures touched my arm, gently, with a soft stirring that felt almost like a caress.

That was when I woke up.

Five a.m., and another strange dream. Typically, I did not remember much about my dreams, but after the surgery I often found weird, vivid images visiting me in the night. I knew this time I would not be going back to sleep; instead I thought about the meaning of what had just paraded through my mind.

A bus, traveling through woodsy scenery — Kal and I were leaving the next day to spend the Memorial Day weekend at a condo in northern Michigan. Snakes — the classic Freudian phallic symbol. It was eight weeks after my surgery, and I was finally allowed to resume sexual activity. The hesitant interaction between me and the serpents — no doubt about it, I was anxious about having sex.

RAMPING UP

During these weeks, I continued to add activities to my schedule.

One that was especially important to me was swimming; the first form of exercise the doctors allowed me to resume. Dr. Andrews, my urologist, was particularly conservative in this regard, because the bladder suspension

~ ~

involved repositioning some of the ligaments that hold the organ in place. He wanted to ensure I had had ample time to heal internally; the jarring associated with jogging, aerobics or even rapid walking led him to forbid any of these pursuits for a full three months. But since swimming does not require any sort of impact, he did allow that form of exercise six weeks after the operation.

As someone accustomed to regular exercise, I had gotten to the point in my recovery that I was starting to miss it. So I headed for the pool.

I was careful getting into the water, not wanting to put undue strain on my still-tender midsection. My first couple of laps were slow and tentative; I was not certain, after so much time off, if I had enough stamina to make it to the other end of the pool.

I was pleasantly surprised. Not only was I able to get from one end to the other without stopping, I ended up swimming nearly forty minutes the first night. I did find that vigorous kicking made my incision area a little uncomfortable, so I simply concentrated on other types of strokes.

I swam twice the first week, and three or four times a week soon after. Like other victories, swimming was an important landmark on my physical and mental journey back to full health.

About this time I also attended my first social function as a full participant. In setting the date for my surgery, I had told Dr. Finn I wanted to be well enough to watch my son stand up as best man at his friend's wedding in mid-May. I also wanted to take candid photographs of the proceedings.

Everything about that evening was absolutely first rate. The bride and groom were glowing. (These were kids my children had grown up with. When did they stop being

~ ~

gawky teenagers and get so mature?) My son was handsome and witty, and I shot four rolls of film. I went home tired but confident everything was okay.

Work, however, supplied a harsh reminder that something major and physical had recently happened to me.

NOT BUSINESS AS USUAL

Getting back to work for real, full-time, where I was spending all day at the office, was just plain tough. I usually was tired even before I got there, merely from getting up, getting ready and navigating the thirty mile home-to-office commute. Fortunately my work load was light after having been gone for so long; my boss was understanding. Typically I would last thirty minutes or so longer each day. By Friday afternoon, after my first five-day week, I was heading home by 4:30 p.m. in full grip of The Shutdown, positively consumed by blinding fatigue.

When my daughter stopped by later, I was short-tempered — I did not want to see her or anybody else. One of the most dramatic characteristics of my bouts with The Shutdown was the box of isolation it erected around me. I simply could not interact with anybody, no matter how hard I might try. At those times, even talking was an effort, as any telephone solicitor who had the misfortune to disturb me found out. I just could not function when The Shutdown descended, as it did many times during my recuperation, and soon enough I learned not to try. When I felt The Shutdown coming, I made my way home as quickly as possible, where I stretched out and rested or slept as much as my body demanded.

~ ~ ~ ~ ~ ~ ~ ~ ~ ~ ~ ~ ~ ~ ~ ~ ~ ~ ~ ~

My level of mental functioning in those days continued to be a matter of concern. As a marketing writer, my stock in trade was my ability to think; instead I found myself unable to remember things I knew I knew — like what ABS stands for (antilock braking system) and how to spell my older grandson's first name. I felt as if familiar words and concepts were obscured by a heavy psychic curtain; I knew what I wanted was back there, but I had difficulty pushing the barrier aside. More than once, I started talking and stopped in mid-sentence, unable to remember where the thought was going. I would intend to do something, then find I could not remember what it was before I could do it. Ideas would start to form, but before I could get them going, they seemed to float away from me. I was scared — what if the ability to think did not come back.

Fortunately, as I demanded more of my brain, it worked better. After once retrieving lost items from behind the curtain, they usually stayed with me. I began to complete my thoughts and feel I was making more intelligent contributions in meetings. I learned to write ideas down quickly before they had a chance to drift away. Within two weeks of my return to work, I had written a short video script and a brief direct mail letter, both of which felt like major accomplishments. More important, I began to regain confidence in myself as a professional, realizing that I could still think and write and be productive.

As I went about my business, I came to realize the heavy achiness in my abdomen as something I was going to have to live with for a while. Strangely, the sensation was not consistent along the entire six inches of the incision; I was always more sensitive on the right end of the cut. The feeling was certainly elusive — one day I would feel almost

~ ~

nothing, the next I was convinced my stomach was dragging down around my knees. I never could discern a clear cause and effect relationship between obvious events like level of physical activity and degree of midsection achiness, even though the heaviness continued for many months.

By now there was an identifiable pattern to my days and weeks. I would start out fairly energetic, feeling like I was functioning at a reasonable level both physically and mentally, then gradually falter as time went on. I tried to do more demanding assignments in the morning or early in the week, when I was still reasonably fresh and sharp, and save routine tasks for later. Eventually, I was able to get through a day and feel reasonably coherent.

I found walking very far, especially up or down stairs, or standing on my feet for an extended period, was difficult and tiring. So I learned to find a chair quickly, and not to apologize for having to sit down. I also took the elevator, if one was available, even when I only needed to navigate a simple flight of stairs. It was weeks before I could wear high heeled shoes comfortably. I tried once or twice when there was a meeting or some other function I needed to look decent for, but I felt unbalanced and my midsection hurt. So I left my heels in the closet and chose flat, comfortable shoes.

One useful trick I used in those early weeks back at the office was the noontime catnap. I would bring a light lunch from home, and at midday drive my car to a nearby parking lot. (Fortunately the company I work for is located in an area where it is safe to do so.) There I would doze for fifteen or twenty minutes, which helped me get through the remainder of the day.

NEVER AGAIN!

Soon enough I was traversing the aisles of the local discount store, stocking up on tissue and makeup and household supplies.

I was busily checking items off my list when I looked up and found myself in the all-too-familiar feminine hygiene section. I had certainly made many emergency trips to purchase these essentials over the years; the amount of money I spent on such supplies would probably have bought me an extended vacation in some exotic locale.

I looked up at the shelves of tampons and sanitary napkins — and started smiling. Next I laughed out loud. The woman going in the opposite direction looked at me strangely, and moved quickly about her business. I actually had to restrain myself from grabbing her and gloating, "I'll never, ever have to buy this stuff again!"

The sense of elation and release keep me floating for days after that incident. Maybe it was beginning to sink in that something very fundamental really had changed for me.

SEX

Kal and I had chosen a lovely setting for our return to physical intimacy, a resort amid the woods and hills of northern Michigan. The time was Memorial Day weekend, lilac season in the North Country, and great bushes of fragrant lilacs were one of my favorite springtime treats.

But my mood was decidedly mixed as we drove northward; I was looking forward to my first weekend excursion

~ ~

since the surgery, and I was also very nervous, knowing that we were about to have sex.

I had been through extended periods of celibacy before, although under different circumstances. Previously, when I had gone without sex, it had been by choice or for lack of a relationship. Medically-enforced celibacy in the context of a close, emotional relationship was another matter entirely, especially since the hiatus had been dictated by surgery that so drastically altered my very femaleness.

So I was worried — had we forgotten how to make love to one another? Would I even want to? Would it hurt? I knew that emotionally we were connected to one another. Could we physically reconnect?

I told Kal about my snake dream as we rolled through the countryside. He agreed with the phallic symbolism, and when I confessed that I was apprehensive, he squeezed my leg and told me with his gentle smile to relax.

We started with a bubble bath. After running a ten-kilometer race that morning, Kal had cramped leg muscles. As he stretched out among the mounds of suds, I rounded the corner of the bathroom with two glasses of wine. Within another minute, I had slipped off my clothes and joined him in the warm tub.

We sipped and talked until the water chilled. Then we toweled off and slipped into bed.

Lovemaking did not come immediately; we snuggled and dozed and talked and then dozed some more.

The most interesting aspect of our conversation centered around the differing responses men and women have to matters relating to the opposite sex's physiology. We women spend endless hours discussing our PMS and our periods and our pregnancies and our sexuality and our partners, often in intricate detail. We generally know much more about the male side of things than vice versa, at least physically. Most men are, at best, reluctant to talk with us about female matters. We, in turn, frequently interpret such reticence as a lack of caring and love. I asked him why men do not want to pay attention to female concerns, especially since they are so important to us.

After saying that he could only answer for himself, Kal replied that for him the apparent disinterest had to do with mystique. Concentrating on the often less-than-pleasant details of female function removed the sense of mystery that he found pleasurable and desirable as part of the sexual act. As he talked, I thought uneasily about the last eight weeks of my life. My surgery and recovery had been anything but glamorous — practical, earthy and painful were the real facts of the experience — and he had been an intimate witness throughout the entire process. Would he, I worried as he slept, find me less desirable as a companion and a lover as a result?

We did get around to making love that afternoon. For Kal, after the long hiatus, that first climax came as an intense release. For me the experience was all right, but far short of a transcendental transport to ecstasy. In fact, it was somewhat uncomfortable, especially the repeated contact against my incision. I adjusted my position slightly to compensate, which helped.

But the physical act *felt* different than I remembered. I did not seem to be as sensitive to stimulation; it took longer and was more difficult for me to get turned on. And the feeling inside was altered; my tissue seemed rigid and uninviting rather than enveloping and soft. When we made love again the following evening, I felt pleasure, certainly, and I enjoyed the physical closeness, but I was not even coming close to climaxing. I worried about the changes, but figured I needed to give it more time.

Part of the difference was that I no longer had a cervix. Now that the prohibition against putting anything inside had lifted, I could explore my vagina with my finger, to see what it felt like.

Empty!

There was nothing in there any more! Instead of reaching in and being stopped by my cervix, I now found a long, unobstructed channel. I could still feel the walls warm around my finger but the cavity did not end anyplace I could feel. That was certainly different from what I was used to. From a sexual standpoint, I knew that my cervix had been sensitive to stimulation; without it and my uterus, would I be able to climax, I wondered, or would the warmth of a climax, starting deep within and spreading outward until it enveloped my entire being, now be just a treasured memory?

It was the third time that the physical magic finally began to rekindle. My climax was a long time coming, and not as intense as I remembered. I seemed to require more clitoral and external stimulation, probably because there was nothing inside to get excited. But it did happen. I cried, with relief that I could still climax, and with gratitude that I could once again experience the pleasure and satisfaction of good sex.

Resuming the sexual aspect of my life had a real quality of relearning attached to it; it was as if that part of me had to reawaken, and get reacquainted with the sensations that were associated with the act. I had expected more of a mountaintop experience, with the breathless excitement

~ ~

typical of a new relationship. Instead, I moved through a gradual reconnecting with that facet of my being. Kal's unfailing love and gentle reassurance helped a lot.

The renewed sexual activity did have a couple of less pleasant, although temporary, side effects: my incision area grew heavier, tighter and more uncomfortable, and I found I had to urinate more often. But those went away shortly, and we got on with enjoying the physical side of our lives.

Even more important than the immediate act was the reassurance that I was still a sexual being, even though my uterus and ovaries were gone.

HOW MEN (AND OTHERS) RESPOND

How hysterectomy affects relationships is a matter of great concern to any woman undergoing this surgery. Although statistics are not available, most women are married at the time of surgery, living as married, or participate in a primary association of some sort. Most have families, and children of various ages, as well. So we wonder, as I did, about how the people most important to us will be affected.

Our most obvious concerns have to do with sex, since removal of the uterus strikes at the core of what defines us as female. These concerns prompt questions that are most difficult to answer, in part because sexual response is so specific and individualized — no two women are stimulated and satisfied in exactly the same way. Beyond sexuality is the issue of how surgery affects relationships in the broader context, since such a fundamental alteration certainly changes us in many important ways.

~ ~

WHAT ABOUT FAMILY RELATIONSHIPS?

The matter of how hysterectomy affects our relationships overall is probably as complex and individualized as people and families are diverse.

Unfortunately, the comprehensive research that might give us clear indicators has not been done.

So we are left, once again, with each other and anecdotal accounts, as the source of wisdom regarding how hysterectomy affects the most important aspects of our lives.

In my own case, my children were concerned with my welfare. After the surgery they helped in every way they could, while continuing to maintain their own commitments to work, school and, in my daughter's case, taking care of her own preschool children. My mom, relatives, friends and coworkers sent cards, flowers, plants, balloons and other small gifts, and called or visited when I felt up to it.

Kal was unfailingly helpful and supportive. He shopped, he cooked, he did laundry, he drove me around — he did all the things I could not, for a period of time, do for myself. He also functioned as my conscience; when I tried to do too much too soon, he pulled me back, insisting I still needed to take it easy. (Generally, he was right.)

In a number of ways, the surgery led to improvements in the quality and depth and character of our relationship. Because I was not able to function in the typical, female manner as the primary organizer, our roles reversed for a time. I appreciated his stepping out of his usual duties and activities to care for my needs, and have told him so, many times. He actually enjoyed this new undertaking, although I am sure he still does not appreciate how extraordinary he

~ ~

really is, and how important a role he played throughout my experience with hysterectomy. (I wish all women were so fortunate.) The forced relaxation softened my typical Type A style a bit, bringing a different dimension to our interaction, allowing his gentler personality to tone mine down. So despite my pre-surgery concerns, things were even better between us than they were before, at least in part because of my improved general health.

Many other women report having similar experiences.

When I asked my mom how my dad responded to her hysterectomy, she described his reaction as very supporting and appreciative. "He was just so relieved I felt stronger and got over my anemia." She went on to say that "sex was better than ever." Since I am old-fashioned enough to feel uncomfortable talking about my parents' sexual relationship, I let that part of the discussion go at that.

Frequently, in my conversations, I heard that men appreciated the positive improvements to the health of the women they loved.

"My husband knew what I was going through," said Alice. "The surgery was a relief for him, almost as much as it was for me."

Sheryl reported a similar experience. "My husband and my family were tired of seeing me feel so bad for so long." Sheryl also felt her surgery came as a relief for those close to her.

Lea felt her husband's attitude helped her throughout her experience. "He was very supportive. He just wanted me to feel better. My kids, too."

Certainly, excessive bleeding, anemia and similar conditions that lead to hysterectomy, affect the entire family, as Helen indicated:

"My horrible PMS and endless periods were impacting the whole family. What a relief when it was gone! My husband, my kids, were confident I'd be totally normal and completely myself again. They didn't hurry me, and they sure took great care of me."

Be advised, however, that these comments, and my experience, apply to surgeries that are normal, recoveries that proceed in a timely manner and after-effects that are not adverse. Severe complications at any point in the process could lead to vastly different outcomes. Much work remains to be done, analyzing the many ways in which hysterectomy can impact family and social structures and interaction.

WHAT ABOUT SEX?

The effect of hysterectomy on sexual response is one of the great uncertainties associated with the operation. Some medical professionals, and women who have had the surgery, contend that removal of the uterus decreases the sensitivity of the labia, clitoris and nipples, as well as precluding the rhythmic contractions of the uterus that some women experience during climax. Removal of the cervix in particular can affect sexual response, since contact with and stimulation of the cervix is often a source of pleasure. Further, loss of the uterus may alter the shape of the vagina and the position of other internal organs. A skillful surgeon will take care to approximate the original length and contours of the vagina, although some loss of length may occur when the uterus is cut away. Inevitably, some nerve damage and scarring of internal tissues also takes place, although, again, a good doctor will keep the loss to a minimum. With all these fundamental changes being made to the body, it stands to reason that sex will be affected in some way.

HERS (Hysterectomy Education Resources and Services) Foundation director Nora Coffey states that of the women she has counseled, loss of sexual feeling has occurred in all of them, whether or not the ovaries were removed.

"Some women have a slight sexual feeling [after hysterectomy]. Orgasm, generally, does not occur. I think you have to consider what sexual feeling was like before surgery, and if you would use the scale of zero to ten, if sex was a ten-plus before, it is likely to be a zero or one after."

That dire warning is enough to scare the heck out of any woman who values her sex life.

On the other side of the debate, many women, and medical people, believe that sexuality is influenced to a far greater extent by emotional, mental and psychological considerations than by physiological structures. They feel that hysterectomy's effect on sexual function is minimal, especially since the vagina, labia, clitoris, nipples and other anatomical structures contain nerves and tissues that respond to stimulation.

I knew from my own experience that I was absolutely sexually responsive, even after losing both my uterus and ovaries. I knew I was reaching climax and achieving sexual satisfaction. Was I just kidding myself, or was sex still a viable, fulfilling aspect of my life?

I turned, once again, to other women's experiences, to gauge their assessments of sex after hysterectomy.

Helen has this to say:

"I was worried that sex would be different. But it wasn't a problem. We cheated by a couple days and made love before the doctor said okay, but there was no discomfort. The sex act felt the same as before. Except now I'm available four weeks a month. That's a real plus. Also, I don't have those awful mood swings any more. So in that sense, sex is even better."

One of the very common side affects of hysterectomy is vaginal dryness, especially for women who also have their ovaries removed. Hormone replacement typically helps alleviate the problem; topical preparations also work. One woman said she had not been told dryness was a possible result of surgery, and wished she had known. "I was extremely dry at first when we started having sex, and uncomfortable. Frankly, it took a while for me to want to again. But now, it's just fine."

Regulating hormones properly can also take a while. "At first I took the standard dosage, and I had zero sexual interest," was how one woman told her story. "I talked to my doctor, and he switched me to a higher dosage of a different drug. After that, my desire came back."

My gynecologist, too, adjusted my hormones about six months after the hysterectomy, adding a pill with a different formulation once a week.

For some women who are still of child-bearing age, hysterectomy can actually bring about a boost in sexual activity and interest. "Not only do I feel so much better, now there's no worry about pregnancy. This is really nice," laughed Alice, in a way that suggested she and her husband were enjoying one another a great deal.

~ ~

The possible negative effects of hysterectomy on relationships, and particularly sex, cannot be lightly dismissed, however. The potential is certainly present, especially if surgery involves removal of the ovaries and the resulting loss of hormones. And while my experience and most of my conversations indicated a positive outcome from surgery, families and marriages can be torn apart.

SO MANY UNKNOWNS

One of the most distressing aspects of hysterectomy is the fact that gauging the long-term effects prior to surgery is virtually impossible. We do not know, and neither does the medical establishment, what will happen to us and our overall health, our relationships, and our sexuality, five years, a decade, four decades after the surgery. These issues are vital, because women typically live many years after surgery. We must go into it understanding there are many unanswered questions.

After the deed is done, there is no turning back. And the lack of good research data to guide us leaves us on our own. Obviously, much work remains to be done in this area. In particular, assessment of the extended psychological, emotional and sexual effects of hysterectomy is long overdue. My treatment in this book of these essential, fundamental and far-reaching issues is brief and superficial at best.

Without good research to guide us, women are left to rely on their own intuition, and the strength and depth of their relationships with husbands, boyfriends, companions, family and friends, in making judgments about the potential affects of hysterectomy on this part of their lives.

Fortunately, women generally find hysterectomy's negative outcomes are temporary, with many indicating positive improvements in their families in general and sex, in particular.

One thing most women can agree on — men apparently do not want to hear or talk about the gory details of what happens to us. Like Kal, they are content to be helpful when we need them, and supportive as we recover. Four of us remarked on that one day over lunch.

Three of the women had undergone hysterectomies; the fourth was experiencing bleeding problems and had recently had a D and C. We were discussing our experiences in graphic detail.

"Do you realize," said one of the women as we munched on soup, salad and sandwiches, "that a bunch of guys could never have this conversation? They are way too squeamish about blood and stuff, unless it's in the abstract, like movies or books. In real life, my boyfriend thinks female problems are repulsive. It's not that he doesn't care about what's happening to me. He just can't handle knowing about it."

We all nodded in recognition, laughed and kept eating, because we knew she was right.

WHAT WAS IMPORTANT

More revelations.

1. Keep being patient! Even though I was getting better, I was far from my old self yet. I had to listen to my body, act accordingly and learn to accept that, and not beat myself up when I had to back off.

2. Do not expect too much too soon. Ramp up activities slowly. In retrospect, I had expected to go into the hospital, have the surgery and after a brief recuperation be back to normal. Not so, in any area, including sex.

3. Expect setbacks; they are part of the process. There were good days and bad days, and I had to learn not to be surprised and frustrated when either occurred.

4. Be realistic is assessing how a hysterectomy will affect family, marriage and relationships. This is the great unknown, and because there is so little information to rely on, I found this even more worrisome than the physical aspects of surgery.

~ ~

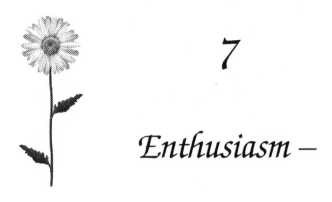

7

Enthusiasm –

Nine Weeks And Beyond

~ ~ ~ ~ ~ ~ ~ ~ ~ ~ ~ ~ ~ ~ ~ ~ ~ ~ ~

Saturday dawned clear and sunny, an early summer day with mild temperatures, low humidity, nothing but sunshine and deep azure sky overhead.

Kal and I woke up early and looked out the window. An ideal morning for a trip to the local farmers market to buy summer flowers and plants. We dressed quickly and were on our way downtown by 7:00 a.m., eager to spruce up the yard for the bright season at hand.

The market was bustling with like-minded shoppers. Enthusiastic vendors competed with one another to convince passersby their petunias would bloom longer and their tomatoes grow bigger than anyone else's. Kal and I pushed our way along through the good-natured crowd, comparing prices and quality as we moved up and down the aisles.

Soon, our arms were loaded with pots and baskets, and we made the first of several trips back to the car to drop our bundles off. Kal left shortly thereafter to attend a meeting, and I was on my own.

Walking back toward the market, I felt the warming sun lighting my hair and soaking into my pallid skin. I crossed the street — and I bounced. I actually skipped. I tipped my head skyward, raised my arms and realized I felt great! I felt tremendous! I felt energetic, optimistic! This day, eight and a half weeks after my hysterectomy, was the first day I felt really, incredibly, amazingly good!

I was buoyant finishing my purchases at the market. I was so peppy I bought more flowers and plants than I had places to put them. I loaded up on cut flowers to spread around the house. I got meat for dinner and fruit and vegetables and anything else that caught my fancy.

I felt good again, and I loved the feeling! I was unbelievably happy and relieved to reconnect with the enthusiastic person I was beginning to fear I had lost.

From the market I went swimming, from swimming to run errands, from errands to planting my flowers, from planting to dressing for a dinner party, from the party, finally, home and to bed.

Sunday was just as full, with spirited lovemaking to start the day, church and a perfectly-timed sermon on optimism, then a Tiger baseball game. I finally ran out of energy late in the afternoon.

By then I was tired, but with the normal sort of tiredness following a busy weekend. I was a little tight in the abdomen after all the activity, but I was walking fully upright and with a welcome spring in my step. Best of all, there was no Shutdown creeping up to grab me.

I was strong! I was joyful! I was finally feeling more like the "me" I liked best!

MORE OF EVERYTHING

That day in early June marked my return to enthusiasm and some semblance of normalcy, with more or less steady progress from there on. I was maintaining a normal work schedule, with evening activities a part of many days. I was busy on weekends, without having to lie down to rest in the middle of whatever I was doing. I was swimming at least three days a week, with running and bicycling added to my list of activities in July. Plus, I was able to keep up with my preschool grandsons, which was an essential test.

Sex was getting better and better. I gradually became more sensitive to stimulation and climaxed with more intensity. There was a slight change in the sensations and the kind of activities that brought me to response, mostly the desire for more external stimulation. On the other hand, I was not bleeding constantly, which increased my interest in sex and my availability.

During one particularly intense week in late June I was able, once again, to reach down and find the reserves of strength I had always depended on. I was used to a fairly hectic schedule, but the events I had to negotiate in that seven-day period were way beyond normal, even for me.

I was in the midst of yet another intense project at the office, with a multi-million dollar piece of business on the line. Then I got the word that an uncle of mine had died in eastern Iowa. In the space of eight days, I flew out to attend

~ ~

the funeral on Saturday, after working at the office from
5:30 a.m. to 7:30 a.m. the morning before the flight; came
back the next afternoon to work until midnight on the
proposal; worked from Monday morning at 8:00 a.m. until
Tuesday morning at 3:00 a.m. to finish the document; flew
out of state on Tuesday afternoon for the presentation to
clients on Wednesday; returned home Wednesday evening;
and left again Friday morning to fly to the other end of Iowa
for my grandmother's 100th birthday celebration. I finally
got home to stay on Sunday, exhausted. But I had made it
through the whole incredible schedule without once facing
The Shutdown, a real triumph for me as I gauged my
progress.

UH, OH

Running late as usual, I hurried to get dressed for
work one morning. Whoops! I stopped in mid-step as I
rushed from closet to bathroom. Darn, there was that
familiar gushing wetness in my crotch. Another period.
Bleeding again.

Simultaneously, I checked my underwear to see how
bad it was this time and reached for the box of sanitary
pads. Then I smiled at myself.

It wasn't blood at all. Kal and I had finished lovemaking a few minutes before, and the drip I felt was left
from that. Not only was I not bleeding, the constant
discharges I had had between periods were also gone.

What I relief! Now a spot of wetness signaled
pleasure, rather than a problem. The realization came as a
surprise that morning, part of the long process of internal-
izing the change in my body. I found that acceptance was

~ ~

gradual; it took time for numerous small events to coalesce into this new reality about me.

NOT QUITE YET

Despite my increased stamina and energy, there were up and down days. At some times I felt like I could do anything. Other occasions found me listless and flat. The abdominal soreness came and went, too; some days I felt nothing at all in my midsection, other times the skin seemed to be stretched so tightly it was hard to my touch.

Other frustrating symptoms continued to make an occasional appearance — most notably, twinges in my bladder area, and thoughts that still floated out of my grasp and away. There were hot flashes, too; not constantly, but most often disturbing my sleep.

I continued to increase my level of physical activity, especially bicycling, in preparation for an extended ride in Iowa in late July. Kal and I did two weekend rides to get ready, the first thirty miles in length and the next fifty. Kal persuaded me that thirty miles was enough for the first outing, and I agreed, under protest. By the time we finished, into a headwind, I had to admit he was right. The day of the second ride was ideal — coolish, sunny and windless. The gently rolling countryside terrain was perfect for bicycling. This time I won and we extended our mileage to fifty. I finished feeling strong, with a real sense of accomplishment. It was important to me to know I could still go the distance, and I had proved to myself that I could.

The ride in Iowa was a family affair, with both my sister and brother coming in from different parts of the country. (Some years earlier our dad had re-introduced all

~ ~

three of us, as adults, to the pleasures of bicycling, and the ride in Iowa had become an annual reunion. In recent years, after his death, we rode in his memory.) Kal and I rode eighty-three miles over two days, enjoying the bucolic scenery and mastering the challenge of several substantial hills. We returned home on Sunday evening and jumped right back into the demands of the work week.

My last experience with The Shutdown came after that bike ride and car trip back and forth to Iowa. I dragged myself through the next three days at work, only to come home and crash before it got dark. Flat and lifeless, I grumbled at colleagues and family. Frustrated, I could not comprehend why I should, once again, feel so drained.

I was worried enough to make an appointment with Dr. Finn; perhaps I had slipped into anemia or hormone imbalance or some other problem I did not know about. She checked me over thoroughly and found nothing wrong. When I described my recent biking excursion, she concluded that had most likely been the culprit in my apparent backsliding. She, once again, counseled patience, and assured me that I was coming along just fine.

Everyone had cautioned me in advance that full recovery would take much longer than I imagined. They mentioned times as long as six to twelve months. I did not believe them, especially because I was healthy and a non-smoker and physically active and not overweight. Now, I had to concede they were probably right.

I had finally come to realize that recuperating moved in the shape of a wave, with constant ups and downs floating along at unpredictable intervals. What I had expected was a steady upward thrust from ground zero, that roared ever higher and never slipped back. I grudgingly came to accept the undulations I experienced, although I was always disappointed when I had a bad day. I was making upward progress to renewed health as the weeks went by, but it was characterized by many peaks and valleys.

To get me over the days when I dragged and drooped and could think only of going to bed, I recalled some advice I had heard from a cross country ski instructor: keep your eyes on the top of the hill. His technique was really quite simple; rather than watching the ground underneath my skis, and thinking about the long, arduous hill looming over me, he urged me to look ahead, to the crest of the hill — concentrating on where I was going, pushing toward easier terrain on the other side.

It worked. On the down days I thought about all the hills I had skied up and over and how much easier the climb always was when I concentrated on the top of the hill. Before long, the slow days came less and less often, and when they did, I could think of them as merely another part of progress toward my goal.

CAPE FLATTERY FOR REAL

We finally got there. In late August, after months of picturing in my mind Kal and me standing on the palisades overlooking the Pacific Ocean, we stood there in fact. Kal was appropriately impressed by the grandeur of the spot.

Being able to share one of my favorite places with him would have been important to me under any circumstances. In this case, I was even more grateful, because I knew how sustaining this image had been in the anxious weeks before the surgery and during the recuperation that followed.

Several times, when The Shutdown was tightly wrapped around me, I had pictured us emerging from the rainforest to admire this stunning vista. Cape Flattery had become a goal for me, one that would mark my full return to health.

Now, we had made it, and I believed the loop was closed.

That was not quite the case.

SIX-MONTH LIFT

The real surprise was the boost in energy I felt six months after my hysterectomy. I had considered myself fully recovered, especially after the excursion to Cape Flattery. Yet, amazingly, in mid-September, I found myself exercising more, running faster, feeling brighter and generally pumped up by an unmistakable surge. The area around my incision was noticeably less rigid, and feeling had returned to the tissue around the cut.

I described these welcome changes during my six-month post-surgery check-up with Dr. Finn in October. First, we shared a laugh when I mentioned I was still finding emergency tampons stuck away in odd places. Medically, she indicated the physical changes around the incision would continue, with more thinning of the scar tissue and increased feeling as the nerves regenerated. The tissue inside, at the top of the vaginal canal, would also soften, as the hardness caused by the layers of stitches corrected itself. My increasing sexual sensitivity was related to the return of feeling high in the vagina, a process she indicated takes six months or more to come about.

Others noticed my improved state. What a lift it was, when a co-worker pulled me aside one day at work and

~ ~

gushed, "You look fabulous! You've never looked better!" All this on a bad hair day when I was not wearing my best colors. She praised my energy level and my positive attitude. She said that other people had noticed and wanted to know my secret.

It was no secret — I had had a hysterectomy.

My friend's praise was a defining moment, one of many I had experienced. This one was especially important because it let me know that those around me had perceived a change for the better. Her comment reinforced both the physical and psychological components that were becoming more pronounced each day.

WE FEEL TERRIFIC!

My feelings of relief and improvement were resoundingly reinforced by many of the women with whom I spoke about hysterectomy. Again and again, I heard phrases like "I feel wonderful!", "It's wonderful everyday," "I feel so much better," "I haven't felt this good in years."

"What a liberation," was how Helen summarized how she felt a year after her surgery. "And what a relief to know I'm really back to normal. There was always a bit of a question during the recovery period.... Will I be healed and healthy?... And now I am. I think back to what it was like when I was bleeding. I tried to pretend nothing was wrong … like most women, I figured 'we gotta carry on' and I carried on. But there *was* something wrong. My quality of life was compromised, and I could not fully enjoy being alive."

When asked if she felt like a victim for having a hysterectomy, as some of the current debate implies, Helen

~ ~

replied emphatically, "I'm not a victim if I'm better after the surgery. And I am so much better. It's like a gift."

Alice echoed those sentiments. "I don't miss any of the problems I had before the surgery. The difference in the quality of how I feel is amazing. I'm still looking forward to finding out what's coming up next."

"Medically, it's the best thing I've ever done," concluded Lea. "I have more energy, I'm not grouchy. I want to grab other women, especially in the feminine protection aisle, and laugh out loud and gloat — never again! I feel so good! I have no doubts having a hysterectomy was the right decision."

I had heard those sentiments before my surgery, from my mother and a number of other women. At that time, they were just words, albeit important reassurance, as I went about making a decision regarding my own circumstances. Now, I, too, had the empirical evidence of my improved condition. I felt so much better, and I knew I would, never again, feel my vitality draining from me.

Having recorded a few of the positive comments from women on the decision to have a hysterectomy, I debated where in this book to place the *Main Women's Health Study* which examined the issues surrounding hysterectomy. I decided it should go here, near the end of my book, because it adds a confirmation to what I and other women, have discovered about the surgery.

THE MAINE WOMEN'S HEALTH STUDY

Published in the April 1994 issue of Obstetrics and Gynecology, *the* Maine Women's Health Study *is*

~ ~

one of the most recent and disciplined medical attempts to look at the effectiveness of hysterectomy in relieving symptoms and improving quality of life. It is an important source for women seeking solid medical information about the surgery, the conditions that might lead to the operation and treatment alternatives for common female problems.

The study is divided into two sections. Part I of the study assesses the effect of hysterectomy for nonmalignant conditions on symptoms and quality of life, and identifies adverse effects one year after surgery. Part II looks at the outcomes of nonsurgical management of leiomyomas (fibroids), abnormal bleeding and chronic pelvic pain.

Two of the authors, Karen J. Carlson and Buell A. Miller, are physicians. The third, Floyd J. Fowler, Jr., is a Ph.D.. All were affiliated with Massachusetts General Hospital and Harvard Medical School at the time of the study. The work was conducted under the auspices of the Maine Medical Assessment Foundation, from June 1989 to January 1991. Subjects were largely white, employed and insured.

In part, the value of the study derives from its methodology. The authors gathered their data from the most authoritative source possible: Women who either had had a hysterectomy (Part I of the study) or who were undergoing treatment for any one of the three most common causes of problems related to the repro-ductive system (Part II). For Part I, a sample of 418 women, ages 25 through 40, were recruited from the practices of 63 physicians performing hysterectomy in the State of Maine. The women were interviewed at the time of surgery, and three, six and twelve months later. This information was supplemented with reports from *physicians and a statewide hospital discharge database. Data collected from patients at the time of surgery included demographic information, gynecologic and medical history, the frequency of symptoms and how much they bothered the patient, the effect of symptoms on quality of life and response to any previous treatment. Postsurgical interviews and questionnaires examined the recuperation process, occurrence of complications, current symptoms and any new symptoms attributable to adverse effects of surgery.*

Part II looked at a sample of 380 women receiving nonsurgical management for fibroids, abnormal bleeding and chronic pelvic pain, as well as 311 women who had hysterectomies as a result of one of those conditions. Eligibility criteria for women treated nonsurgically were designed to identify women with conditions that could also be treated by hysterectomy.

Specifically, women studied in Part II were eligible when fibroid tumors produced uterine size equivalent to eight weeks gestation or greater; women who complained of abnormal bleeding were checked to eliminate malignancy as a cause; and women with chronic pelvic pain had to exhibit the condition for at least six prior months, and have undergone laparoscopy to rule out endometriosis, malignancy or other conditions warranting specific treatments. Eligible women were interviewed at the onset of treatment, and at three, six and twelve month intervals. In addition to demographic information and gynecologic and medical history and treatment, the authors looked at the effect of symptoms on quality of life as measured by subjects' ratings of degree of discomfort, limitation in activity, worry related to the condition and an index of how they felt about their symptoms.

Study results for Part I showed the most frequent causes of hysterectomy among the sample to be fibroids (35%), abnormal bleeding (22%) and chronic pelvic pain (18%). Other diagnoses included endometriosis (10%), cervical intraepithelial neoplasia (7%), pelvic inflammatory disease (1%), and others (2%). In one third of the cases, the physician reported multiple diagnoses. The majority of women interviewed reported some or a lot of discomfort or limitation of activity related to their pre-operative conditions. Eighty-eight percent of the women studied had had children, and 34% were capable of bearing children at the time of surgery.

For the conditions described, hysterectomy resulted in marked and statistically significant improvements in a range of symptoms, including pelvic pain, urinary symptoms, abdominal swelling, fatigue, psychological symptoms and sexual dysfunction. There was no difference in symptom relief at three and twelve months between abdominal (73% of the sample) versus vaginal (27%) hysterectomy and between hysterectomy with bilateral salpingo-oophorectomy (removal of the tubes and ovaries) and hysterectomy without removal of the tubes and ovaries.

However, hysterectomy was not universally effective in eliminating symptoms documented prior to surgery. Obviously, bleeding problems were eliminated, but pelvic pain persisted in 5% of patients twelve months after surgery, problems with urination continued among 9% and fatigue persisted in 20%. Adverse effects — new problems not reported before surgery — also occurred. The most frequent were

~ ~

weight gain (reported by 12%), and hot flashes (13%). Also reported were feeling depressed (8%) or anxious (6%), and problems with diminished sexual interest (7%). Hot flashes were most common among women who had their ovaries removed; 91% of such women began hormone replacement therapy soon after surgery. For all adverse symptom measures, a greater number of patients reported problems at either six or twelve months following surgery and not at both intervals. This suggests that a single assessment of post-hysterectomy problems may result in over-reporting some symptoms that are temporary.

In other words, although long-term adverse effects of hysterectomy have been suggested in other sources, this study indicates the development of new physical and psychological symptoms in women who did not demonstrate such symptoms prior to hysterectomy was infrequent. (The fact that this study limited the follow-up period to one year could ultimately affect longer-term results. This work has not been done at that time.)

That hysterectomy entails a significant period of recuperation was well supported in the study. Seventy-two percent of women reported post-operative pain, lasting a median period of 14 days. Ninety-one percent felt fatigue for a median of 21 days; 35% continued to experience fatigue at three months. The median length of time before working at the usual level among women who worked outside the home was 42 days. Overall, three months after surgery, 72% of women felt their general health was much better.

The core finding in this study related to responses to the question: "How would you feel if you were told you were going to spend the rest of your life feeling the way you have for the past month or so — your symptoms would be no better and no worse." Before hysterectomy, 76% of the sample said they would be "unhappy, terrible" with that situation. After surgery, in response to the same question, 75% said they were "pleased, delighted." In other words, the women involved in this study demonstrated that, for a wide range of conditions, hysterectomy resulted in a marked improvement in quality of life.

Study results for Part II, which assessed the effects of nonsurgical treatments for fibroids, abnormal bleeding and chronic pelvic pain, attempted to add to the virtually non-existent literature in this area, providing useful information that can be used to guide clinical decision making.

Management of symptoms was accomplished through a variety of treatments. Women with fibroids were treated through simple observation of symptoms, nonsteroidal anti-inflammatory agents, iron or hormone therapy. Those in the abnormal bleeding group received hormone therapy, a D & C, iron and other non-hormone treatments. Patients with chronic pelvic pain received various nonsteroidal agents, hormone therapy or merely observation of symptoms.

Medical therapies, especially for abnormal bleeding and chronic pelvic pain produced statistically and clinically significant reductions in symptom levels for some women at three months, which were sustained at twelve months. Relief of symptoms was also associated with improvements in some measures of quality of life.

However, one-quarter of the women treated nonsurgically at the outset of the study had undergone a hysterectomy after one year of follow-up; this was particularly true for women with severe fibroids and those with multiple diagnoses. In addition, an appreciable number of women receiving medical therapy (25% of those with abnormal bleeding and 50% of those with chronic pain) continued to report their symptoms were a "medium" or "big" problem after a year of treatment.

The data suggests that conventional medical therapies represented in this study are ineffective in some patients. At the same time, women demonstrating asymptomatic or mildly symptomatic fibroids reported little change in either symptoms or quality of life.

One unexpected outcome of this study was an association between higher educational level and nonsurgical management of all conditions represented. The higher educational level was also an important predictor of a positive treatment outcome in patients treated nonsurgically for abnormal bleeding and chronic pelvic pain.

P.S.

"You're well-ironed now," commented the Red Cross nurse as we watched a drop of my blood sink quickly to the bottom of the test medium. I had gone in to make my first post-hysterectomy blood donation, seven months after the surgery. This time, I passed the hemoglobin screening in no uncertain terms, in contrast to previous rejections for low iron in my blood.

As we discussed my recent medical history, I described how much better I felt. The nurse also had had a hysterectomy, which gave us a basis for instant rapport.

"I know exactly what you're talking about," she affirmed. "Before you have it, it's like your entire psyche gets focused on the bleeding."

I certainly knew what that was like.

"That's the only thing you can think about, because it preoccupies you all the time."

I was well-acquainted with that feeling, too. It was what she said next, with a broad smile, that really connected.

"Then, it's such a relief. Your whole outlook changes. Afterwards," she concluded, "It's a whole new world!"

WHAT WAS IMPORTANT

Additional revelations.

1. Expect ups and down. Once I realized recovery is a wave, it was easier to deal with the reoccurring peaks and valleys. I had expected steady progress upward, and that was not at all the way it occurred.

2. Keep your eyes on the goal. I found the focus-eyes-on-the-top-of-the-hill technique helpful at this point. I learned to keep my thoughts on the goal of feeling better. Then, the process of getting there was easier and more pleasant, and seemed to happen with less effort.

3. Get as much information as possible. I found myself frequently wishing I had known more about what to expect during surgery and recovery. More detailed information about the entire, prolonged process would have helped me understand that I was getting healthier than I had been in a long time.

4. Enjoy feeling better. It takes a while, but it is great when it comes.

Part III

How To Thrive

Taking time to reflect on the hysterectomy process helps put it all together. This is not an experience to be taken lightly, yet understandings beyond the obvious may result.

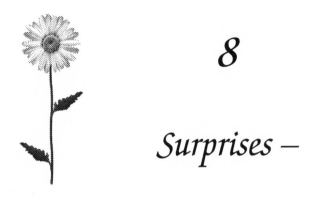

8

Surprises —

Things To Watch Out For

~ ~

In seeking to synthesize my entire experience with hysterectomy, I have isolated a number of issues I would like to share as points of caution. In addition to my recollections, I have added observations garnered from other women who have had the surgery.

These are not health-related concerns so much as commentaries about several of the more subtle ramifications that may accrue from the extended hysterectomy process, before, during and after any actual surgery may take place.

With that said, let me detail several items that women want to watch out for.

~ ~ ~ ~ ~ ~ ~ ~ ~ ~ ~ ~ ~ ~ ~ ~ ~ ~ ~ ~

FEELINGS OF TURMOIL, HESITATION AND UNCERTAINTY

I have spent many pages in this book describing the difficulty I had in making the decision to have a hysterectomy. I wavered, I vacillated, I hesitated, I got hysterical, I felt isolated and very much alone as I attempted to gather the facts needed to make an intelligent, informed decision about myself.

To other women who may feel the same sense of agitation, and wonder, as I did, what in the heck happened to their usual take-charge ability to deal with whatever happens, I want to say two things: first, don't be surprised if you have that experience, and second — it's not you!

You are not imagining that what you read and hear is contradictory. You are not alone in feeling that your doctor may not be giving you much guidance — or recommending surgery you don't want. You are not the first woman, nor, unfortunately, the last, to wish there were some easy solution to your female problems.

Unfortunately, confusion is the situation we have on our hands. Deciding to have, or not to have, a hysterectomy, is not an easy choice, and certainly not a clearcut one.

So hang in there! Keep looking for and insisting on as much information as you find helpful, and then trust your intuition to help you make the choice that is right for you.

A SENSE OF DISORIENTATION

If you do choose to have the surgery, plan on feeling disoriented for a while. Although I was told by my doctor

~ ~

and others to expect an extended period of recovery, I was not prepared for how bad I felt in the two weeks after surgery, the power of The Shutdown that descended on me over and over again, or the frustration I felt when I wanted to be healthy sooner than I was able.

Beyond the physical symptoms, I was unnerved by feeling so out of sync with myself and my surroundings. For a person who generally regards herself as well-grounded in practical reality, I found the disorientation and sense of disruption tough to deal with.

Looking back, I still feel as if there is a gap in my sense of alignment, a abyss in my orientation with the world covering April and May of 1994.

To other women undergoing hysterectomy, I can only say, be realistic, both about the physical pain connected with the surgery and the length of time you will need to return to full function. There will be a shift in your universe for a while, so expect that. The good news is, it will pass.

THE ABSOLUTE FINALITY OF NO MORE CHILDREN

I can honestly say this was not an issue for me, but a number of women I spoke with, especially those under the age of 40, took pause at the finality of hysterectomy. Frequently, they said their reactions surprised even them, especially because they assumed their families were complete.

The issue was not that they wanted to have more children. But by having a hysterectomy, they forever precluded the possibility of choice. Often, they felt increased sympathy for childless women, understanding in

~ ~

a new way the desperation women feel who want to have children and cannot.

Fortunately, hysterectomy among young women who want to bear children is not common, and myomectomy may provide an option if children are desired. The problems that most commonly lead to hysterectomy, like fibroids, tend to increase in severity as women age, and presumably are finished bearing children. As one medical professional pointed out, women who undergo hysterectomy before having the children they want, generally do so for grave medical reasons. In those cases, the central issue may be saving the patient's life.

Nonetheless, in the matter of child bearing, hysterectomy is absolutely final. Every woman must understand that, and the effect such knowledge may have on her, in no uncertain terms. Confronting one's feelings about having children is an issue every woman contemplating hysterectomy must address.

MENOPAUSE SURPRISE

Several women who kept their ovaries brought this to my attention, and I include the discussion because it certainly counts as one of those things to watch out for.

As I have described, I had my ovaries removed, putting me into immediate menopause. I expected that and counteracted by taking synthetic hormones.

But women who kept their ovaries had a different experience. They were surprised by menopause.

"I sort of forgot about it," was how Donna, who had a hysterectomy in her mid-forties, described what happened to her. "All of a sudden I started having hot flashes and vaginal dryness and got real grouchy and had trouble concentrating. At first I didn't realize what was going on. Then my gynecologist reminded me that, at 50, I was exhibiting symptoms typical of menopause. Without my periods to warn me, the whole thing really snuck up on me."

Sheryl said the same thing. "I was still smoking in those days, so I went into menopause early, when I was 42 or 43. (She had had her hysterectomy at 33.) "I had hot flashes and night sweats, my interest in sex went down to zero — I really worried something awful was wrong with me." Her doctor put her on synthetic hormones, which smoothed out her symptoms and soon had her feeling like her old self again. Still, the advent of her menopause came as a jolt.

Obviously, a woman who has a hysterectomy and keeps her ovaries will still experience menopause. But as these women, and others, reported, it may seem to appear without warning, with no uterus and no changes in periods to serve notice.

Both Donna and Sheryl advised doctors to pay more attention to menopause in women who have had hysterectomies. They agreed that their doctors should have monitored them more carefully, and prepared them better for the inevitable onset of the change of life.

THE "ROUTINE" MYTH

Again and again, I saw, and still see, references to hysterectomy as "routine surgery." In terms of technique, difficulty and frequency, from a medical perspective, that may be true. But such characterizations contributed to my underestimating how involved the hysterectomy process

~ ~

really proved to be. As a woman who has now traversed this territory, I must take issue with this wording. I know, now, that having a hysterectomy is a major life experience. The process needs to be treated with a lot more seriousness and respect than it often receives.

FAILURE OF THE PROCEDURE

Sometimes, surgery just does not work, and women agreeing to an operation must be advised of that possibility. Failure is not frequent, but it does happen.

Such was the case with one women I interviewed, who had a hysterectomy in association with a bladder suspension. The hysterectomy was indicated because of chronic pelvic pain, and she welcomed the end of that problem. It was the bladder suspension, which was the primary reason for her surgery, that was not successful:

"I waited a number of years before I finally had this done, and all that time nobody told me much of anything. They sure didn't tell me going in that the success rate with bladder suspensions is only about eighty percent. I thought this would all be over and done with after the surgery, all the leaking and urinary problems I'd had for so long.

"My post-surgery complications started while I was still in the hospital. I got a bad infection; I knew I had it because I'd had so many before, but it took the doctor a couple days to believe me. Finally, he put me on an antibiotic, but by then I could barely control myself and I was really in pain. It's been eight or nine months since the surgery, and I'm still on pills to control my urine. The surgery was not

~ ~ ~ ~ ~ ~ ~ ~ ~ ~ ~ ~ ~ ~ ~ ~ ~ ~ ~ ~

successful. I finally changed urologists, because I totally lost faith in my old doctor. I'd go in for an appointment and he wouldn't even examine me, just take a urine sample and tell me sometimes it took six months for a suspension to kick in. The new guy says there's only a thirty to forty percent chance he can help me. I'm so disappointed, and so frustrated things aren't better than they are."

This story, even though it focuses on bladder suspension rather than hysterectomy, underscores that surgery is definitely a risk. Things do go wrong, procedures can be less than completely successful and the patient may be left with a problem that cannot be solved.

LOSS OF CONTROL OF ONE'S OWN BODY

The possible long-term consequences of hysterectomy are illustrated by the experience of another woman, who had surgery ten years ago, in her mid-thirties. Prolonged pain and heavy bleeding led to the removal of her uterus and ovaries.

"I was prepared for my uterus being taken out. Then, as I was being wheeled into surgery, the doctor told me they were taking out my ovaries, too. Afterwards, I cried for a year. I was not prepared for the psychological sense of loss I felt at something being taken from my body. Within three months I was on anti-depressants, and of course, hormones. I started on the hormones right after the surgery, first pills, then the patch, then shots, then back to the patch. Yes, I was bleeding heavily before the surgery, but at least it was my own body doing it to me. Now, I have to depend on a patch on my hip to regulate my body. I feel a definite loss of control. I'm trying homeopathic treatments and Chinese herbs, something totally different, to get myself regulated. I finally got my anemia fixed using those techniques. The next thing is to get off the anti-depressants, and eventually I want to end the hormones, too. As for the surgery, I'm angry at the loss of control of my own body and at the failure to explore other treatments for my bleeding. So, yes, I regret having it done."

Clearly, the negative consequences of hysterectomy, both physical and emotional, can be far more serious than the temporary problems I experienced. Let me stress, once again, it is not an act to be taken lightly.

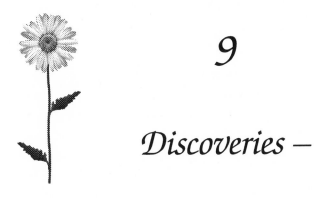

9

Discoveries –

Unexpected Lessons Learned

~ ~ ~ ~ ~ ~ ~ ~ ~ ~ ~ ~ ~ ~ ~ ~ ~ ~ ~ ~

I expected my surgery to relieve my protracted bleeding and other symptoms, which it did. For that I am extremely grateful.

Beyond the obvious improvement in my physical condition, I found myself making other discoveries along the way. Other women reported similar experiences. So I wish to share our realizations, as a way of adding depth and texture to the journey we have been on.

LITTLE PLEASURES

I want to mention a couple things I did not miss during the recovery period, and count as positive aspects of the experience.

First was the long commute to the office and the time and expense associated with the daily drive. Obviously, when I went back to work, I had to resume commuting, but I quickly came to appreciate how nice it was to do without that hassle, at least for a while.

Then there was the rushing. Like most of us, I frequently pursue a too-busy schedule that has me feeling pressed and late much of the time. I enjoyed the respite from rushing and have tried to hang on to some of that mellowness even after I was fully back to my old life.

As I felt stronger, the opportunity to lunch with friends I do not see very often was a real pleasure. As I was recuperating, these pleasant occasions were a welcome break in my days, and they were an important part of my feeling like I was returning to the land of the vital and alive.

MEDICAL LESSONS

In the course of my research, I interviewed several medical professionals, who to a one, were surprised by their experiences on the patient side of the medical equation.

Jody is a surgical nurse:

"Being on the flip side of what I do was very educational, and more than a little scary. I was surprised by my fears, for example. Try as I might, I couldn't make light of them. Now, I take the fears of my patients a lot more seriously than I did before.

"The feeling of being the patient was humbling. As a medical professional, I was trained to disassociate myself from the patient; the patient is a body and that's it. Now, it was my body, and I was almost humiliated by the lack of modesty and dignity I was allowed. Being spread-eagled in front of the doctor and the nurse and who knows how many others is very embarrassing. I'm a lot more aware of what that feels like, and I try to be more sensitive to my patients as a result."

Helen is the nurse in charge of a women's unit at a medium-sized hospital:

"Of course I knew what was happening from a clinical standpoint, but my hysterectomy was the first time I experienced what it felt like to be the patient. I had misgivings about what I was feeling, at how long it took me to recover, about how I'd feel eventually. I'm thinking now, on the other side of the surgery, about starting a hysterectomy support group at the hospital to help women make decisions and also to aid them through the whole experience."

Lynn admitted that, as a physician, suddenly being the patient was eye-opening, and humbling:

"The first thing they wanted to do at the hospital was take my glasses away. I'm absolutely blind without them, so I refused to give them up, and ended up keeping them with me in the operating room. They do the same thing to patients who wear hearing aids. Taking away the glasses or hearing aid removes the patient's contact with reality. That's not fair. It increases fear rather than diminishing it. Then, when the anesthesiologist couldn't get the needle in for the epidural on the first stick (Lynn remained conscious throughout her surgery, as described in Chapter Four), he wouldn't fess up that he was having trouble. I knew better, but they tried to tell me otherwise. After the surgery, I was very interested in the quality of nursing care at the hospital. I know I received kid glove treatment, because they do that for physicians. But I could sure see room for improvement, especially in handling things like shift change. Care basically shuts down for forty-five minutes during shift change; and that's not in the best interest of the patients."

Reflecting on her experience, Lynn talked about the nature of the hysterectomy process:

"Gynecology is so invasive, and so personal. I think many of the younger gynecologists, both men and women, realize that, and are less patriarchal than previous generations. But I was still surprised that I had to demand to participate in decision-making. I had to insist on options in order to get them. Other women must do the same."

We can only hope, as patients, that our doctors listen to Lynn's advice and follow it. As she indicated, and I learned, women must watch out for their own best interests. We must demand all the information available and insist on treatment that is right for us.

INTERNALIZATION TAKES A WHILE

During the many years that I was fighting my symptoms, I adjusted my routines and life style to accommodate the facts of that reality. I have recounted the disruptions and compromises and subterfuges I made in order to carry on with my life.

By the same token, it took about six months after the surgery for me to undo all those prior years and construct new patterns of doing things.

~ ~

There were the little things, like not leaking when I sneezed or constantly checking my panties to see if I was bleeding again. For many weeks I found myself reverting to old assumptions. Gradually such incidents accumulated to form a revised reality, but this process of internalization did not happen overnight.

Once the fundamental nature of the changes sank in, I began to realize that a transformation had taken place beyond the mere cessation of my symptoms.

I felt liberated! Getting rid of my long-standing problem had given rise to a tremendous sense of elation! A consuming preoccupation was removed, forever, from my life.

In its place was a new sense of vitality. I felt connected with depths of energy that had been hidden from me. I felt more focused and more creative. And I felt more pleasure at being a woman than I had in many years.

As I spoke with other women, most echoed my sentiments. Once over the hump on recovery, fatigue, sex, hormones, work and all the other associated considerations, women reported tremendous improvement after their hysterectomies, not just in their physical health, but in all areas of their lives. It is worth noting that of the women I interviewed, half had undergone surgery at least ten, and in several cases more than twenty, years prior to our conversation. Perhaps dispelling some of the concerns regarding long-term adverse effects, most of these women continued to state emphatically that for them hysterectomy had been the right choice.

Trudy described her feelings this way:

"Solving this long-standing physical drain gave me a freedom about my life and routine I

~ ~

hadn't had in a long time. I knew I could plan to do something and be up to doing it. Not bleeding gave me so much more energy; that increase in energy has been a great gift. Bleeding was always the downside of my femininity. Now I feel freer in a lot of ways to be who I am."

Trudy's observations touch on one of the core issues surrounding hysterectomy — without my uterus, am I still a woman?

I never had the slightest doubt about that part of the experience. I *knew* I was still a woman, because my sense of self and self-worth was never tied to my ability to bear children.

My mom's assessment was even more to the point. "Nope, I never felt blue."

"Who are these people?" asked both Donna and Sheryl, when confronted with the femininity question. "Maybe their support at home is lacking. Or maybe they don't have anything else going on in their lives." Both insisted hysterectomy had absolutely no affect on their womanliness. In fact, like Trudy, they felt more positive about themselves after the surgery than before.

"There's so much negative material out there about hysterectomy," they continued. "It's time to hear from all the women who know, without a doubt, that the surgery improved the quality of their lives."

Lea brought another slant to the matter. "I don't care how much the naysayers dump on hysterectomy. I'm stronger. I'm more in control. There was no other choice for me."

Perhaps Alice put it most succinctly:

"I didn't know people were supposed to feel this good!"

CHANGING TIMES

Despite feeling, so often, that I was left to muddle through hysterectomy on my own, I have found encouraging hints that changes may be coming.

Women's health issues, in general, are becoming the focus of increased attention, both from the medical community and from society at large. A procedure as common, and as controversial, as hysterectomy will surely benefit from such examination.

One hopeful effort is the Women's Health Initiative, a $628 million study being conducted by the National Institutes of Health. In an attempt to redress the historic shortfall in research on women's health, this project will examine many of the issues of concern specifically to women. Unfortunately the results won't be available until 2005, which is too late to help anyone faced with an immediate problem. But at least something is finally happening, and that is an encouraging sign.

Perhaps clearer guidelines for women struggling with the hysterectomy decision will emerge from the investigation. Perhaps more information will become available to let women know what they might expect at every phase of the process. Perhaps we will feel more supported in our choices. Hopefully, medical science will find better ways of dealing with bleeding, fibroids, endometriosis, pelvic pain and other conditions, making surgery, ultimately, unnecessary. To get there, we must step up the pressure, demanding the research, analysis, inquiry and discussion that can give us the answers, and alternatives, we need.

Meanwhile, we must seek more openness in the medical community to the specialized needs of women and ask for greater participation with our doctors in making decisions about our health. So fundamental a choice as hysterectomy must never again be made by a physician who approaches the uterus with a cavalier "you don't need it anymore, take it out" attitude. Every woman, who so much as hears the word "hysterectomy" uttered in her presence, must be absolutely certain *she* has made the choice of her own volition, because she is convinced surgery is the best alternative for her.

10

Insights –

Going Forward

~ ~ ~ ~ ~ ~ ~ ~ ~ ~ ~ ~ ~ ~ ~ ~ ~ ~ ~ ~

Throughout this narrative, I have referred to my experience with hysterectomy as a journey. It has indeed been that, and in many ways.

The physical saga has been the most fundamental component of my experience, and I have detailed that side of the process throughout this book. But there has been more to my journey than cutting and extracting and healing, crucial though those have been.

It has come as a great surprise to me that this has been an important period of personal growth.

I have learned worthwhile things about myself, my family, my relationships, my work and my life. I have gained increased sensitivity to the world around me. I am paying more attention to goals and priorities and, as a result, I am making some adjustments.

I might have embarked upon such a period of reflection even without the surgery, since reassessing one's world and place in it is a common occurrence for someone who has reached, as I have, the half-century mark. On the other hand, the forced inactivity and extended recuperation afforded me an excellent opportunity for contemplation. Whatever the impetus, I believe I am and will continue to be a better, more satisfied person as a result.

GREATER APPRECIATION

"Life can be short." "Appreciate the moment." "Pursue your dreams." "Today is the first day of the rest of your life."

I have paid as much lip service over the years to those familiar shibboleths as anyone else; now, I actually believe them.

By putting me so graphically in touch with the physical side of my persona, the hysterectomy reminded me that unexpected things, illnesses, accidents, unforeseen tragedies, do sometimes happen to people. Coupled with such events as older colleagues retiring, elderly relatives dying and the occasional acquaintance struck down by circumstance, I came to realize, with new depth, that now is, indeed, a time to be savored.

The pain of surgery, followed by the miracle of recovery, illustrated in an extremely personal way that my body, is, at one and the same time, a fragile temple and a tough, resilient vessel. The hysterectomy process also brought to my attention the emotional side of my persona,

~ ~

revealing depths of power and passion that I may not have known I possessed. Reducing the complexities of physical and mental processes to their most elemental functions, as surgery did for me, led to a deeper appreciation that the body/mind complex is an absolutely astounding phenomenon. As such, it must be cared for and cherished in every way and at all times. I believe I have always held the miracle of life and personality in high regard. Now, at the risk of sounding overly dramatic, I find myself approaching these with increased reverence, even awe.

As a result of my surgery, I believe that I take my life and good fortune a little less for granted, especially the bounties of a strong body, mental acuity and a sound night's sleep. For the first time ever, my surgery forced me to grapple with the millstone of ill health, and I did not like it. I had the advantage of knowing I would get better, even though there were days when I found that hard to believe. I admire those who must deal with real disease or permanent disability, and thank God daily for the gift of good health.

LETTING GO

To say that I have felt I had to "do it all" is a fair assessment of my approach to living. In many ways, as a long-time self-supporting single woman and single parent, that was not far off the mark.

Suddenly, after the hysterectomy, I could not conduct myself in the manner I had been accustomed to for most of my adult life. I could not be in control of everything. I couldn't shoulder all the burdens of my children and my house and my finances. I could not be the primary organizer and caregiver in my relationship. For a while, I could not even drive a car.

The lesson was a very important one for me: it's okay to be vulnerable and hurting. It's okay to ask for help. Amazingly, when I was finally forced to stop being all things to everybody, people responded. My children, my family, Kal, my friends — all were not only willing, but eager and pleased to rise to the occasion. That realization, working in tandem with the physical restrictions, has prompted me to be easier on myself in general. That I could let up a little, did not have to push so hard all the time, take the time I needed for me — all were among the more subtle outcomes of my surgery.

Once I relaxed and let go, I discovered a "me" that was more agreeable, more mellow, more easy going and perhaps, easier to get along with. I realized I liked the feeling, and decided to hang on to it.

Because I had to ask for help when I needed it, I find that I am now more willing to speak up about other wants and needs. In the work setting I am more apt to seek mutually-negotiated solutions than simply imposing my will. In general, I believe I make more of an effort to reach out to others, having reaped the rewards of having others reach out to me. Naturally, old habits remain with me, making my move to greater mellowness and increased conciliation work better some days than others. But the lesson remains with me, and I have a revised notion of ways in which I want to conduct my life.

~ ~

THE WORK ETHIC

Forcibly removing work from my frame of reference, even for a five week period, led me to reflect on both the positives and negatives associated with this essential activity.

On the one hand, I quickly realized how crucial work is as a source of organization — it tells us when to rise and retire, where and how to spend our days and nights and, to a large extent, what to think about. Work has always been important to me, especially since I come from the sturdy Midwestern stock that used their strong arms and broad backs to build this country. I have long known work to be more than a necessary source of income; it has also served me as a source of achievement and confidence and pride.

During the weeks when I was not working, I came to realize the difficulty of ordering one's life without the structure afforded by the work model. As with so many other aspects of my hysterectomy experience, I was lucky; I never missed a paycheck. And I knew I had a good job to go back to, one that I truly enjoyed. At the same time, I found myself thinking about so many others not afforded the security of knowing they can support themselves and their families, especially in the face of illness. And in a broader context, I wondered how it is that people acquire the work ethic, especially when they do not see it in operation as children or surrounding them in their daily lives. I also realized how devastating the lack of such basic skills must be, both on a personal level and for society as a whole.

But there was another side to not working, the one that brought me to understand how much work preoccupies me,

~ ~

how often it becomes the driving force in my life. I found that without work to talk about, worry over, glory in and otherwise demand my attention, I had time to think about what else might be important. I believe I learned something about putting work in its proper place.

That has led me to seeking a better sense of balance among the various aspects of my life. I am not about to stop working, even if some unforeseen financial windfall were to make it forever unnecessary; on the other hand, I am protective of my time for other activities. I am trying to put my work in perspective as crucial and rewarding, without allowing it to be the consuming force in my life.

STRONGER RELATIONSHIPS

I am enjoying stronger associations since my surgery, with my children, my friends, my colleagues and, yes, the man in my life. The reasons probably can be attributed to a number of factors, many related to what I perceive to be the increased openness in myself and a more relaxed approach to living. I also believe I have come to appreciate the value and importance of all my various relationships more, and I am more willing to share my thankfulness with the people who mean the most to me.

As I have recounted, my relationship with Kal, in particular, has deepened. We were able to share a dimension that heretofore we had not encountered together, and happily, our mutual participation in my surgery and recovery proved to be a plus. We spent a great deal of time together, especially during the first month of my recuperation. Kal became the primary caregiver, while I could do little else but accept his generosity. In the process, we both

~ ~

discovered yet another facet of the other's personality, which led us to appreciate and love one another even more.

STRENGTHENED CAMARADERIE

I learned, once again, and with new power, that we women are our own best friends.

We must continue to turn to one another for information about such fundamental life choices as hysterectomy. We must ask and share openly our own experiences as a means of helping other women as they pass by the same way.

I found other women to be my most valuable source of knowledge and comfort throughout my hysterectomy experience. Whether these women had undergone the surgery, were contemplating it, had decided against it, or were friends, co-workers, health care providers or concerned strangers, they were unfailingly understanding and supportive of me.

I hope other women will find the same kind of understanding and compassion. Because when it comes to so personal and powerful an experience as hysterectomy, we need one another.

SO MUCH TO BE THANKFUL FOR

In seeking to put the hysterectomy experience in perspective, I have to say, using the typical clichés, that my life to this point has been a mixture of ups and downs, pain and pleasure, highs and lows. Although I have had to work hard for what I have accomplished, I have been blessed with

~ ~

the tools I needed to move forward. Like most of us, on occasion I have been visited by substantial disappointments, which have been balanced by many gifts. I have terrific children, exceptional grandchildren (aren't everybody's), wonderful friends, a rewarding job and a great relationship. And now, I have a freshened perspective on life.

Hysterectomy taught me, in a new way, that I have much to appreciate and be thankful for. Always, I count my many, many blessings. I will continue to do so every day for the rest of my life.

FINAL THOUGHTS

Hysterectomy is serious business — invasive, painful, prolonged and scary.

I went into my hysterectomy with a positive attitude and the clear conviction that this surgery was the best alternative for me. Now, from the vantage point of one who's been there, I must emphasize that hysterectomy cannot be taken lightly. I would never recommend that a woman undergo this surgery without strong medical indication that it is the best course of action. The experience is just too difficult and too physically challenging to be anything other than a last resort.

On the other side of that, I have to say —

I feel terrific!

I also feel incredible! sensational! superb! tremendous! magnificent! marvelous! glorious! and any other superlative I can dream up. No amount of hyperbole can adequately describe how much better I feel.

I am now able to enjoy belonging to the female half of the species more than I have in many years. I am no longer

~ ~ ~ ~ ~ ~ ~ ~ ~ ~ ~ ~ ~ ~ ~ ~ ~ ~ ~ ~

dragged down by the negative consequences of being a woman, which makes me feel even more feminine than I did before.

The changes I have experienced as a result of my hysterectomy extend far beyond the mere absence of bleeding. My entire personality is brighter, stronger, healthier. I am a happier, more optimistic individual. I am more productive. I am more energetic. I am, in just about every way I can imagine, a better "me."

What hysterectomy did for me, and for most other woman I have talked to, is provide a tremendous sense of relief. An enormous burden has been lifted from my psyche, and I have emerged into an expanded acceptance and appreciation of myself.

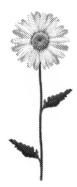

Epilogue –

Bonus!

~ ~ ~ ~ ~ ~ ~ ~ ~ ~ ~ ~ ~ ~ ~ ~ ~ ~ ~ ~

Exactly one year later, Kal and I were back at the same northern Michigan ski resort where my countdown to hysterectomy had really begun.

The day was, once again, glorious, with clear blue skies and perfectly groomed crosscountry ski trails. I moved enthusiastically up hill and down, recalling the episode that had pushed me to reconsider my "no, never" position on the operation, and taking stock of my post-hysterectomy condition.

I knew I felt better than I had in a long time; I even felt like I was skiing with more energy and stamina than I had the year before. I had gained back the five pounds I had lost, but not much more. The horror stories I had heard about women sinking into depression or ballooning up or losing all interest in sex had not materialized. I was taking synthetic hormones with no discernible side effects. And my profile had certainly improved. With my enlarged uterus gone, if I stood up really straight and pulled my hips back and sucked in like crazy, my stomach was almost flat. But since I was a long way past sleek-bodied adolescence, I really did not mind. The scar marking my incision had slowly turned from red to white, and it was neither glaring nor obvious; instead it looked like a crease in my skin.

From time to time, my lower abdomen still got tight and heavy around the incision, often when I was on my feet more than usual; in fact, I could feel the sensation developing that day as I skied. But I had gotten used to the occasional coming and going of the phenomenon, so it did not bother me much anymore. I did have to admit I'd lost one sometimes-useful item along with my uterus — my convenient excuse. Now, when I was ill-tempered or bitchy or draggy or otherwise unpleasant, I could no longer blame it on another episode of "This Thing" or anemia or PMS.

Emotionally, I felt stronger and more together. My relationship with Kal had not only survived, it had taken on new depth and meaning. My children, grandchildren and friends also benefited from my improved health. Professionally, my work was better and more focused; I had more attention and energy to put into it. All in all, I had to conclude that the hysterectomy had brought about marked improvements in virtually every area of my life.

Given my positive feelings, I reflected on a question I had been asked several times: Why did I wait so long?

I could easily isolate a couple of factors. One had to do with financial back-up. As the sole support of myself and my two children for nearly two decades, I had always been

~ ~ ~ ~ ~ ~ ~ ~ ~ ~ ~ ~ ~ ~ ~ ~ ~ ~ ~ ~

conscious of financial security. If my income were to be cut off (as it had been a couple of times through job losses) there was no one for us to fall back on. Now, at long last, I had accumulated a bit of a financial cushion, and my children were finally old enough to take care of themselves.

I thought about Kal and the pleasant weekend we were spending together. That led me to consider the matter of emotional support. Certainly, I would have had the backing of family and friends had I had the hysterectomy sooner. Kal's contribution was another matter. My concerns regarding the effects of surgery on our relationship were deep and very real. At the same time, his willingness to help me sort out the issues before the operation, and his unfailing love and caring throughout the entire process, were (and are) a tremendous source of strength. I might have decided to have the hysterectomy without him, but having him as part of my life made it easier to take action.

All analysis aside, the best answer I could come up with as to why I did not do it sooner was an old standby: It just wasn't time. First, the many pieces that make up my life had to get aligned properly. Then, and only then, my intuition told me it was okay to go ahead.

I smiled to myself as I passed the very spot on the trail where my long-standing bleeding had manifested itself so dramatically a year earlier. As if to emphasize, "Hey, I don't need you anymore!" I put on an extra burst of speed when the hut where I had sought shelter came into view. On this gorgeous day, I was enjoying myself immensely, especially since I knew I would never have to worry about dripping blood in the snow again.

~ ~

After several hours of skiing and thinking, I headed back toward our condo, feeling both pleasantly tired after a hard workout and cheered by the fine day and my vitality. I spotted a man and woman coming toward me on the trail who looked vaguely familiar. As I got closer I could see it was Gene and Jenny, people I knew from the running group I attended downstate.

"Hey, hi, great day!" I called as I pulled to a stop. "What are you guys doing up here?"

"Sue, guess what! I've got fifty bucks for you in my car!" was the first thing Jenny said.

I was astonished. "Wow! Why! I'll take it, but how come?"

"You won the Super Bowl pool!"

I vaguely remembered putting a couple of dollars into the pot sometime before the game. I promptly forgot all about it, because I never won anything.

We met at her car, and I triumphantly collected my winnings. Then I headed back to the condo to tell Kal; skis over my shoulder, a crisp $50 bill in my hand.

I felt like this was a final benediction on my long struggle. This time, I *had* won, and in so many ways.

Sources

American Medical Association Encyclopedia of Medicine. Clayman, Charles B., ed. New York: Random House, 1989.

Anstett, Patricia. "Delicate Decisions." *Detroit Free Press,* March 8, 1994.

Anstett, Patricia. "Read All About It: Woman Survives Menopause." *Detroit Free Press,* May 26, 1992.

Anstett, Patricia. "You and Your Hormones." *Detroit Free Press,* December 13, 1994.

Arnot, Bob. "Finding the Right Medical Care Can Mean the Difference Between Life and Death." *Good Housekeeping,* vol. 216, no. 1, January 1993.

Atkins, Andrea. "The Take-Charge Patient. (The Woman As Partner in Health Care Decision-Making)." *Ladies' Home Journal,* vol. 107, no. 11, November 1990.

Bakos, Susan Crain. "The Operation I Didn't Have (Hysterectomy)." *Ladies' Home Journal,* vol. 110, no. 11, November 1993.

Bernstein, Steven J., et al. "The Appropriateness of Hysterectomy, A Comparison Of Care In Seven Health Plans." *Journal Of The American Medical Association,* vol. 269, no. 18, May 12, 1993.

Bickell, Nina A., et al. "Gynecologists, Sex, Clinical Beliefs, and Hysterectomy Rates." *American Journal Of Public Health,* vol. 84, no. 10, October 1994.

Brody, Jane E. "The M Word." *New York Times,* reprinted in the *Detroit Free Press,* May 26, 1992.

Brody, Jane E. "Vitamins, Herbs and Exercise May Ease Menopausal Symptoms." *New York Times,* reprinted in the *Detroit Free Press,* May 26, 1992.

Carlson, Karen J.; Nichols, David H.; Schiff, Isaac. "Indications for Hysterectomy." *The New England Journal of Medicine,* vol. 328, no. 12, March 25, 1993.

Carlson, Karen J.; Miller, Buell A.; Fowler, Floyd J. Jr. "The Maine Women's Health Study: I. Outcomes of Hysterectomy." *Obstetrics and Gynecology,* vol. 83, no. 4, April 1994.

Carlson, Karen J.; Miller, Buell A.; Fowler, Floyd J. Jr. "The Maine Women's Health Study: II. Outcomes of Nonsurgical Management of Leiomyomas, Abnormal Bleeding and Chronic Pelvic Pain." *Obstetrics and Gynecology,* vol. 83, no. 4, April 1994.

Cassidy, Jane. "Aborted Hopes. (Patient Consent to Operations Such as Abortion and Hysterectomy)." *Nursing Times,* vol. 89, no. 41, October 13, 1993.

Charles, Allan G. "The Hysterectomy Hoax (book review)." *Journal of the American Medical Association,* vol. 272, no. 3, July 20, 1994.

Christmas, Rachel Jackson; Warner, Virginia Williams; Johnson, Pamela. "Fibroids: A Report." *Essence,* vol. 24, no. 9, January 1994.

Cutler, Winnifred B. *Hysterectomy: Before and After.* New York: Harper Perennial, 1990.

Demmerstein, Lorraine; Wood, Carl; Westmore, Ann. *Hysterectomy, New Options and Advances.* Melbourne: Oxford University Press Australia, 1995.

"Dilation and Curettage." *American College of Obstetricians and Gynecologists,* March 1992.

Dranov, Paula. "Curing Fibroids Without Hysterectomy." *Good Housekeeping,* vol. 214, no. 6, June 1992.

Dranov, Paula. "When the Diagnosis is Fibroids: New Treatments Will Prevent Hysterectomy for Millions of Women." *American Health,* vol. 12, no. 7, September 1993.

Elias, Marilyn. "Estrogen May Cut Women's Alzheimer's Risk." *USA Today,* November 20, 1995.

Emling, Shelley. "Women Seek Out Female Gynecologists, But They Face A Long Wait." *Detroit Free Press,* August 15, 1994.

"Estrogen After Hysterectomy." *Consumer Reports,* vol. 57, no. 5, May 1992.

"Every Woman For Herself." *Newsweek,* May 25, 1992.

"Fibroid Tumors Need Not Be Treated." *HealthFacts,* vol. 17, no. 162, November 1992.

~ ~

Friedman, Andrew J.; Haas, Susan T. "Should Uterine Size Be An Indication For Surgical Intervention In Women With Myomas?" *American Journal of Obstetrics and Gynecology.*, vol. 168, no. 3, March 1993.

Gagnon, Ria. "Doctor, Please Help Me! (Posthysterectomy Syndrome)." *Ladies' Home Journal,* vol. 106, no. 4, April 1989.

Grimes, David A. "Shifting Indications for Hysterectomy: Nature, Nurture, or Neither?" *The Lancet,* vol. 344, no. 8938, December 17, 1994.

Good Morning, America, Show #2181. Interview with Dr. Stanley West and Dr. Michelle Battistini, October 21, 1994.

Hackman, Brian. "There's No Place Like Home. (Surgeon's View of Early Discharge of Hysterectomy Patients)." *Nursing Times,* vol. 89, no. 37, September 15, 1993.

HERS Newsletter. Interview with Dr. Howard Posner and Nora W. Coffey. vol. 2, no. 4. (date unknown)

"Hysterectomy Hesitation. (Alternatives to Hysterectomy)." *Harvard Health Letter,* vol. 19, no. 2, December 1993.

"Hysterectomy and Its Alternatives." *Consumer Reports,* vol. 55, no. 9, September 1990.

"Hysterectomy and Its Alternatives: One Small Step Toward Assessing the Options." *HealthFacts,* vol. 19, no. 180, May 1994.

"Hysterectomy, When Surgery Is the Solution." *American College of Obstetricians and Gynecologists,* September 1991.

Huckshorn, Kristin. "Hysterectomy Alternative Generates Debate." *Detroit Free Press,* February 12, 1992

Hufnagel, Vicki. *No More Hysterectomies.* Penguin Books, 1989.

"Important Facts About Endometriosis." *American College of Obstetricians and Gynecologists,* March 1991.

"Loss Of Ovaries May Raise Heart Disease Risk." Body And Mind, *Detroit Free Press,* November 21, 1995.

"Menopause." *Newsweek,* May 25, 1992.

The Merck Manual of Diagnosis and Therapy. Berkow, Robert, ed. Merck Sharp and Dohme Research Laboratories, 1987.

~ ~

"Most Hysterectomies Not Worth It." *Special Delivery,* vol. 16, no. 2, Spring 1993.

Nakhnikian, Elsie. "Heading Off Hysterectomy." *Health,* May/June 1992.

Nechas, Eileen; Foley, Denise. *Unequal Treatment.* New York: Simon & Schuster, 1994.

Neerbaard, Lauran. "Think Young Before Making Decision on Hysterectomy." *Detroit News,* date unknown.

Payer, Lynn. "The Operation Every Woman Should Question." *McCall's,* vol. 122, no. 9, June 1995.

"Pelvic Support Problems." *American College of Obstetricians and Gynecologists,* March 1991.

Ravn, Pernille; Lind, Charlotte; Nilas, Lisbeth. "Lack of Influence Of Simple Premenopausal Hysterectomy On Bone Mass And Bone Metabolism." *American Journal of Obstetrics and Gynecology,* vol. 172, no. 3, March 1995.

"A Real Midlife Crisis." *Newsweek,* June 26, 1995.

Rothberg, Lee. "Hysterectomy: The Shocking Truth." *Woman's Newsletter,* Issue #54. (date unknown)

Schofield, M. J.; Bennett, A.; Redman, S.; Walters, W.A.W.; Sanson-Fisher, R.W. "Self-reported Long-term Outcomes of Hysterectomy." *British Journal of Obstetrics and Gynecology,* vol. 98, no. 11, November 1991.

Sheehy, Gail. *The Silent Passage: Menopause.* New York: Random House, 1991.

Shelemay, Kay Kaufman. *A Song of Longing.* Urbana and Chicago: University of Illinois Press, 1991.

Strausz, Ivan. *You Don't Need A Hysterectomy.* Addison-Wesly Publishing Co., 1993.

"Study Tracks Hysterectomies. (Unnecessary Surgery Can Be Prevented Through Patient Advocacy)". *Cancer Researcher Weekly,* November 7, 1994.

Summit, Robert L., Jr.; Stovall, Thomas G.; Lipscomb, Gary H.; Washburn, Scott A.; Ling, Frank W. "Outpatient Hysterectomy: Determinants of Discharge and Rehospitalization in 133 Patients." *American Journal of Obstetrics and Gynecology,* vol. 171, no. 6, December 1994.

"Understanding Hysterectomy." *American College of Obstetricians and Gynecologists,* September 1991.

~ ~

"Unnecessary Hysterectomy: The Controversy That Will Not Die." *HealthFacts,* vol. 18, no. 170, July 1993.

"Uterine Fibroids." *American College of Obstetricians and Gynecologists,* January 1994.

Wallis, Claudia. "The Estrogen Dilemma." *Time,* June 26, 1995.

Warrick,Pamela. Feminists And Medical Establishment Wage Battle Over Menopause." *Detroit News,* August 14, 1994.

Weathers, Rosemary. "Is Hormone Replacement Therapy Okay? It All Depends On The Woman." *Detroit News,* July 13, 1995.

West, Stanley; Dranov, Paula. *The Hysterectomy Hoax.* New York: Doubleday, 1994.

Wilbanks, George. "Ovarian Cyst Riskier After Menopause." *Detroit Free Press,* July 11, 1995.

Wiltz, Teresa. "Hysterectomy Hysteria. (Avoiding Unnecessary Surgery)." *Essence,* vol. 23, no. 6, October 1992.

Zonis, Nadia. "The Laparscope Revolution. (Laparoscopy in Hysterectomies and Reduction of Fibroid Tumors)." *Ladies' Home Journal,* vol. 109, no. 6, June 1992.

Afterword

To every woman, and most especially those in any phase of the hysterectomy experience — may you enjoy vast happiness and abundant good health!

The author welcomes comments.
Please send correspondence to :

S. E. Barber
c/o BookPartners, Inc.
P.O. Box 922
Wilsonville, Oregon 97070

To order additional copies of

Hysterectomy:
Woman To Woman

Please send _____ copies at $14.95 for each book, plus $3.50 shipping and handling for the first book, $2 for each additional book in the same order.

Enclosed is my check or money order of $_____
or [ ] Visa   [ ] MasterCard
#_____ Exp. Date ____/____
Signature _____

Name _____
Street Address _____
City _____
State _____ Zip _____
Phone _____

(Advise if recipient and shipping address are different from above.)

For credit card orders call:
1-800-895-7323

or

Return this order form to:

BookPartners

P.O. Box 922
Wilsonville, OR 97070

NOTES

Use this space to record your thoughts, and especially issues to discuss with your doctor.

_____

_____

_____

_____

_____

_____

_____

_____

_____

_____

_____

_____

_____

_____

_____

_____

_____

_____

_____

_____

_____

_____

NOTES

NOTES